Praise for
UNDERBELLY

'*Underbelly* invites us all down the rabbit hole into the
wild, weird and sometimes wonderful corners of the
Internet. I raced through it'
EMMA GANNON

'Darkly voyeuristic – but with heart'
GRAZIA

'I don't think I've ever turned the pages of a book
so quickly. This is the first book I've read that really
captures life online – the satire is so sharp, but the
emotional core of the story is so tender and pulsing.
Truly excellent storytelling'
DAISY BUCHANAN

'Captures the depth and complexity of female
relationships under the glare of social media'
STYLIST

'I barely breathed in the last few pages. This is more
than a page-turner, it's unputdownable, it will stay with
you long after the last page. I've never read a book that
so perfectly encapsulates the complexity – and belly-
laughing heart – of female relationships'
CHERRY HEALEY

Anna Whitehouse is the fiction-writing pseudonym for Anna Whitehouse and Matt Farquharson. Together, they are the co-authors of *Sunday Times* bestsellers *Parenting the Sh*t Out of Life* and *Where's My Happy Ending?* They are both journalists, co-founders of the website Mother Pukka and the Flex Appeal campaign to have flexible working enshrined as a legal right for all. Anna also presents a weekly show on Heart Radio. *Underbelly* is their first novel.

This book contains references to domestic abuse, self-harm and baby loss.

UNDER BELLY

ANNA WHITEHOUSE

ORION

First published in Great Britain in 2021 by Orion Books,
This paperback edition published in 2022 by Orion Fiction
an imprint of The Orion Publishing Group Ltd
Carmelite House, 50 Victoria Embankment
London EC4Y 0DZ

An Hachette UK Company

1 3 5 7 9 10 8 6 4 2

A CIP catalogue record for this book is
available from the British Library.

ISBN (Mass Market Paperback) 978 1 3987 0248 6
ISBN (eBook) 978 1 3987 0249 3

Typeset by Input Data Services Ltd, Somerset

Printed and bound in Great Britain by Clays Ltd, Elcograf S.p.A.

MIX
Paper from
responsible sources
FSC® C104740

www.orionbooks.co.uk

For our girls.

PROLOGUE

THE HOSPITAL

Four and a half years ago, somewhere upstairs in this hospital, they cut a baby out of me. The doctor was tall and had a voice so deep it sounded like every word was sinking to the floor. I was with him for exactly twenty-seven minutes, and in that time he sliced through my womb and said reassuring things that he must have said a hundred times before, calm as a man tying his shoelaces.

He pulled out my baby and the nurses did their checks while I was there with my legs and belly wide open.

The walls were peach, with yellow hazard signs: wash this, dispose of that, be careful of those. I can't remember much else because the drugs were coursing through my veins. The doctor walked up to my end, smiled, said 'congratulations' and left, because it was someone else's job to do the stitching up and either he had another baby to set free or he just wanted his lunch.

And now I'm in A&E and my life is about to end.

When they do the first incision for a Caesarean, a little arc of blood shoots up in the air. They don't tell you that, because you

1

can't see it past the sheet they hang above your chest. And you don't feel it, because of the anaesthetic. But I did hear it: a little patter of three or four drops, like water spilled on a plastic mat.

And now I wonder how many pints of blood a person needs and if she has enough left.

The waiting room is full of grey faces and tired nurses, none made happier by the plastic Santa on the main desk. A man comes in wearing overalls and dust, with kitchen roll around his arm and blood slowly seeping through the layers while his wife applies more. A woman in a headscarf is bent double, moaning gently in the corner, willing whatever pain she is in to go away. There's a young boy in a football kit with his kneecap in the wrong place and his mum is stroking his head as he tries not to cry.

This is where people land before a nurse can see them, or where you have to wait if you arrive with a victim. A kind of medical purgatory.

The lights are too bright and I feel like an animal in here, like I'm being checked for ticks. The hospital smells of illness and the heating is on too high. It's the perfect place for germs to breed and there's a ball of dust and hair tumbling around in the corner of one of the air vents, looking for an escape. That vent is making us sick.

My hand closes around my phone, but my phone is dead and my heart jangles.

If they take one pint at blood donations and that leaves people needing a biscuit, then more than two is probably bad.

And there was so much blood. More blood than you'd think one woman could hold.

The machine-gun flutter starts in my heart again, like an old, toy rattle wildly shaken until it stops dead, and I wonder when will the police come and what will they say when I don't have any answers.

This is what I'll be known for now. There will be before today and the moment I became a killer. It feels like my ribs are pushing inwards, all the air is rushing out of me and I can't get it back in quick enough. And I'm tapping my phone against my chin because I want to know what the signs of a heart attack are, but mostly because I want to know what they're saying about me.

I want to tell them that she made this happen. I want them to know that it's her fault. Because it is. It really is.

But it won't matter because they'll come for me anyway. There will be thousands by morning. They will hear my name all over the world and they won't be happy until I'm dead too, so I might as well get on with it.

FOUR MONTHS EARLIER ...

1

LATE AUGUST

LO

I'm looking in the mirror. My left breast hangs slightly lower than my right. What were once pert grapefruits stare back at me like socks weighed down with tennis balls. Each nip points in a different direction, one towards Scout's room, the other to the laundry basket.

At school, you'd put a HB pencil under your boobs in the bogs. The Pencil Test. There was no traction back then and the pencil would fall to the ground. Now I could stash a Crayola set under there.

I hoist them into a bobbled bra and wrestle myself into yesterday's leggings. It's an undignified process where I squat like a Zumba teacher until Lycra meets crotch.

'Scout, you ready?' I holler, while pulling a sweatshirt over my messy curls.

There's silence.

'Scout?'

Further silence.

'Scout, we've got to get a move on,' I say, a bit more militant.

'YES,' she huffs, like a tiny teenager.

She's four. It's a fleeting insight of what's to come.

I go to her room and her toy box is upended. She's surrounded by debris and looks like someone on day three of a festival. I tiptoe through the Lego to straighten her up and am glad that she still needs me.

'One more minute, OK? Then breakfast. Porridge, OK? With a honey "S" on it?'

She looks up at me with those big Bambi eyes, nods and re-enters her imaginary world.

My knees creak in unison with the stairs as I walk down past black-and-white family photos. Johno and I on our wedding day, our happiness spilling out of the frame; Scout, Johno and me on Brighton Pier; my dad holding Scout like she's a rugby ball. A collage of our lives, missing out the grey bits in between that bind these moments like grouting.

I put her porridge in the microwave. I've got two minutes and I swipe to my Instagram profile: @the__lo__down__:

Lo Knox
Campaigner
Get your tits out for the . . . baby. Making room for
breastfeeding at work.

I scroll right back to the beginning of my feed like it's going to hold the key for what to share with 32,567 people today. There's a post of Scout's plate with a ketchup smiley face, two peas for eyes and a soggy fish-finger nose: 'Raising a smile #friyay' – and another of a badly cropped quote I've stolen off the internet: 'May your coffee be strong and your Mondays short.'

The worst is a photo of me and my friend Amara, with a caption that reads: 'Never a dull moment with this one' – which was, if I'm honest, fairly dull. I've known Amara since day one at Oakley Comp, and I still love seeing her, like a kid loves Haribos, even if it doesn't happen that much anymore. The caption doesn't do our twenty-three-year friendship justice.

I want to delete these early ones, but people will notice. There are a few that pick up every detail, like they're in the wings just waiting for you to go off script so they can message: 'Oh, didn't you say you were off the booze?' – with a screen grab of an opened bottle of wine in my kitchen. Even when you're sleeping, someone is watching.

Last night's post has gone down OK. It was me, collapsed on the sofa, head to toe in 'minimalist lifewear' from new Scandi label Etisk. They're my main client, and their stuff is OK, if a bit 'greige' – the colour of a pair of knickers you've had since 2001. But Etisk pays the bills and feels like progress from my first ad, for bog roll, which saw me praising the three ply like it was a silken glove.

Somehow it's been ten minutes and we need to get a move on.

'Scout, BREAKFAST.'

Silence.

'Scout, your porridge is *on* the table.'

I say this like stating the location will spur a pre-schooler into action.

'Scout, come on, please don't make me come upstairs.'

I instantly hate my tone.

'Scout, don't make me come upstairs.'

I hear a rustle, but then silence again.

'Right, I'm going to count to three and if you're not downstairs . . .' I tail off, unable to find a suitable threat. 'One, two . . .'

I start thundering upstairs and hear a clatter of Lego as she appears at the door, beaming impishly.

*

I hold Scout's shoulders, guiding her to the porridge on the kitchen table as though she might escape. Period pains that have been building since I woke pulse more urgently. Once she sits down, I open what Johno calls 'the kitchen drawer of shame', a dumping ground for everything that doesn't have a place. It's deep and cluttered, and as I scrabble for pain relief, a pair of toy-rabbit ears clatter to the ground. I pop two tablets, rub my stomach gently and check the time: its 9.20 a.m. She's still eating but we need to leave. However much time we have, I always seem to be rushing.

We don't use the buggy anymore, so that Scout can run and climb and skip wherever we go, but it means every journey takes twice as long. I ask her to put on her shoes and coat, knowing she's not really capable of doing either, and I run up-stairs two steps at a time to have a panic wee. Like a child, I always need to go just before exiting the building.

I pee and flush, wash my hands and take a moment for the mirror. My hair is wild, my mahogany curls jutting out at odd angles, and as I run my hand through them, a few strands come away, a lingering pregnancy gift. It's supposed to stop after the first twelve months, but I still shed like a Labrador in summer.

I dust blusher onto the apples of my cheeks and look slightly clownish but more alive. My eyes are bloodshot, tiny capillaries gathering to remind me of late-night Netflix and early-morning shoulder taps from Scout.

I wonder if this frenzy will intensify when she starts Reception next week.

I come down to find she has her shoes on the wrong feet and is wearing her pillar-box red coat like a cape. Her skin is like porcelain, so perfect it looks filtered, and her eyes are bright with life. She looks like a proud elf and I just want to scoop her up and absorb her, but we don't have the time.

'Nugget! You ready to fly?'

'Yes.'

She raises up her arms to make her coat flap.

'OK, let's just fix your shoes.'

'Why?'

'They're on the wrong feet!'

I say this like it's wonderful. Like it's charming and she's amazing, because she knew all along, and I give her a full smile. Then I squat on one knee to swap the shoes over.

'Sometimes I wonder if my shoes are the wrong way round or my feet are.'

'Yeah!'

She accepts this as fact. Adults also get their shoes on the wrong feet and she has no reason to feel ashamed.

I pull on my bright yellow mac as our front door slams behind us. This coat is what Johno might call 'a bold choice', but the colour always lifts my mood.

I suck in air. The sky is grey and heavy, but there's a freshness, a little hint of autumn in late summer. We make good progress for five minutes before Scout becomes distracted by someone's front hedge. We're on a street of little Victorian terraces, two-beds mostly and half of those chopped into flats, and I take the chance to pop another ibuprofen. Scout doesn't ask what I'm doing because she's looking for the perfect leaf. Normally, if she sees me take something, she wants to know what it is, because in her world, silver foil only covers sweets, and I think she likes the scratching sound or that little pop when the pills come out of their pod. Johno's convinced she's going to accidentally overdose one day, because I sometimes leave things within reach.

'I'm serious,' he says, like I'm the child.

But today Scout is pulling a deep green privet leaf from someone's hedge. She gently puts the leaf in the palm of her hand like it has feelings and needs to be looked after. I often find leaves, twigs and ring pulls in her bedside drawer at home. Once there was a small bone (a sparrow? A mouse? Louisiana fried chicken?). These things are a little band of misfits united by a kindly four-year-old.

I watch Scout pluck another leaf and put it in her pocket. She does a half-skip and asks if she can walk on a crumbling white wall. I never stop her from climbing, but I like that she asks. It's safe adventuring. She's wearing new thick-soled boots that look like they're from an army-surplus store. Her legs look like stalks poking out of soil bags.

There's a girl at nursery who stamped on Scout's feet a few weeks ago, and when I picked her up, all tear-stained, I asked her what she thought we should do. Instead of 'tell the teacher,' she said, 'get bigger boots,' and she's barely taken them off since.

My first ever negative comment on Instagram was about Scout – *Why do you dress her like a builder? It's cruel. Let girls be girls.*

I remember reading 'cruel' and feeling pins and needles flutter across my chest. I wanted to say, 'Let Scout be Scout,' but I stopped myself, because I didn't want to argue with a stranger about my daughter's dungarees.

I look back at my phone. The flurry of likes and comments warms something inside me, like that feeling you get when a stranger asks where you got your dress. You're embarrassed by the exchange but secretly glad they asked because it makes you walk a little taller. The likes cut through the banal: the meal planning, the running out of foil, the Hoover-bag replacing, the toast-crumb sweeping, the dentist booking. Then a quick boost, a flutter of someone's approval and a flood of agreement and I feel something, like I am someone with a purpose. It's ridiculous because I have Scout, and she is purpose enough.

I once had dreams of being an author but ended up chasing an algorithm. I did write press releases for employment law firm, Darby Cooper, but they made me redundant six months after I returned from maternity leave. I fought them and lost, so now I fight online. But fighting doesn't pay the bills like androgynous culottes and bog roll do.

Scout shouts for help and pulls me away from my phone. I have a vague idea that it's the second time she's called. She's climbed onto a wall that's missing a few bricks and has found herself stranded at a rusty gate and a crumbling precipice. I scoop her up and swing her round until her face lights up with glee. She leans into me as we walk along the pavement, weeds fighting their way through cracks, to Little Tykes Nursery.

The single-storey building has visible steel girders and uniform red bricks. It's right next to a B-road, but there's a leisure centre next door with five-a-side courts where the kids sometimes go to play on rainy days. Inside, it smells of bleach and nappies. Outside, it's fag butts and petrol fumes.

I'm ten minutes past the nine-thirty cut-off, after which you're supposed to call ahead. There are no other stragglers as I ring the bell, wait to be recognised, then pull the door open and hurry Scout down the grey vinyl-floored corridor, decked with its paintings of smiling farmyard animals. Scout's key worker, Karla, comes out of the classroom and Scout gallops towards her with an enthusiasm that fills me with equal measures of joy and jealousy.

Whenever I'm struggling to get her out the door because she's refusing vital outerwear, I say, 'But we're going to see Karla,' and that usually calms her down.

She boomerangs back to me and I give her a peck on her head.

'Love you, have a great day.'

'Love you.'

Then I wave to her back as she strides into the classroom in her big boots.

It feels like a lifetime ago that she was burrowing into my underarm as a baby, not wanting me to leave on those mornings when I, too, couldn't say goodbye. I remember sitting on the steps of the leisure centre next door during her settling-in week four years ago. I cried a little, my face going blotchy, but then had to lurch on into a legal world that doesn't show emotion.

I wonder what I'll do when Scout starts school next week.

A cramp sears through my stomach and brings me back to the present and my forehead beads with sweat. It's hot in here. The kind of sticky heat only found in nurseries and old people's homes. There's a smell of nearly burnt toast in the air that makes me want to eat even though I'm not hungry, but it's mixed with the faint scent of nappies, which makes me want to gag. I feel like I'm in a very colourful Petri dish. I can hear the kids in one of the classrooms singing 'Baby Shark' at top volume. There's a late-fee warning on the noticeboard, alongside a dozen 'turkeys' whose bodies are brown handprints squashed onto paper.

I rub my stomach, wondering if I can make it to the toilets at Asda, but it's a fifteen-minute walk. I'm late for my period and this is Mother Nature's penance. The kids' loos are open, so I peek inside, seeing the familiar low saloon doors in their bright colours, each stall with a different cartoon vehicle painted on it. I've spent an unhealthy amount of time in here negotiating with Scout to wee before we leave each evening.

Just as I'm about to duck into the stall, I'm interrupted by Danni, the manager, heading down the corridor hand-in-hand with a toddler. She's a stern woman who has a strict policy of not smiling.

'Is there a loo?' I ask her.

'You can't go in there.'

'I know, but is there one for grown-ups?'

She stares at me as if I'm hiding a chisel and plan to march off down the high road clutching the cistern.

'The only other toilet is for staff,' she says.

'Do you mind if I use it?'

For a moment it feels like I might have to tell her what my plans are.

'If you really need to,' she says.

She points at a red door that I always thought was a cleaning cupboard.

'It's in there.'

'Thanks.'

I smile, head through the door, close and lock it, and instantly nausea washes over me from belly to throat. It feels as if a gerbil is scrabbling around in my uterus and I think I might be sick. I pull my yellow coat off, drag my leggings down and sit, my thighs spilling over the toilet seat. There's a mop and bucket in the corner and enough bright blue bleach to scrub down an oil tanker. Stuck to a peeling full-length mirror on the back of the door is a poster with a council hotline and the headline: 'ACCUSATIONS AGAINST YOUR STAFF?'

I can just hear Danni ushering the toddler to the loos down the corridor. I feel oddly guilty on this toilet, like I'm breaking the law by being semi-clothed near other people's children. One class is singing about a turtle and they reach a crescendo at the end of each verse with a screeching 'POP'. The smell of toast and nappies has somehow managed to seep under the door and I feel as if I'm about to retch, the cramps making me curl over.

I look down at my pants and they're patched with blood. My tailbone aches. Then something passes through my vulva, like a little bar of soap slipping out of a hand. I stand up, stare into the pan and see a familiar dark oval bundle, enveloped in a veiny sac.

I want to flush it away.

But I can't stop looking at the bloody mass, the size of a 5p coin. The water goes pink. I stand there for ten seconds or ten minutes. Tears well and slowly creep down my face as I process being pregnant once again and losing that little life in the same moment.

Children's laughter ricochets around the corridor outside. I turn, catching sight of myself in the mirror and I'm standing with my leggings around my ankles, my yellow coat on the floor. Under the brash lighting, I look grey. Grey, dimpled thighs, flecks of grey hair among the dry, brown curls and a grey sheen to my skin. My eyes are hollow. I stare at my C-section scar, a little pocket of flesh hanging over it like an overburdened bag-for-life.

I sit back down on the toilet seat and sobs build, making my shoulders shudder. I want to be at home. I want to be in a warm bath, or hidden beneath a duvet, not perched above an unviable foetus in a nursery toilet. I want someone to look after me.

I breathe slowly, focusing on the soft hum of electricity coming from the strip lighting on the ceiling. I pull at the long roll of toilet paper and wipe myself over and over, until there's just a rose-tinted residue on the tissue. I stuff my pants with a large wad of paper and pull up my leggings as I stand and wash my hands in the sink.

I stare back into the toilet water. It's so small and for a moment I want to hold it in my hands. But it is so tiny and incomplete, there is nothing to hold. Just dead cells and blood and an ending.

I flush. Pink water fades away. The most inhumane funeral.

I don't want to look in the mirror again, but I need to wipe away my mascara stains. I take a foundation stick from my coat pocket, drag it across my cheeks, chin and forehead and roughly blend it into my salty, dampened skin. I have the pallor of a Tudor milkmaid, but I dust bronzer across my cheeks to come back to the twenty-first century.

I pull on my yellow mac, step out of the toilet and Danni is standing there.

'Mum! No phones in the facility please!'

'Ah, yes, sorry.'

I didn't even realise it was in my hand and slip it away again. She looks at me a bit longer.

'Are you all right, Mum?'

I've been coming here for years, but they still call me 'Mum' because it's easier than remembering my name. It always makes me feel like another sow in the farmyard.

'Fine! Thanks for the loo!'

And to stop her worrying, I throw out a huge smile.

My skin feels clammy as I step out of the nursery. The air chills the sweat on my skin. I want to call Johno but can't bear waiting for him to work out what to say. He will go silent, and say he's so sorry, and then he'll go silent again.

I call the health centre and hold my phone to my ear, careful to avoid the thin crack that runs across one corner of the screen. It rings three times and then some music kicks in: a panpipe version of 'Ain't No Mountain High Enough', which is a new tune for them. A robotic female voice tells me I am fourth in the queue.

Transit vans and skip carriers shoot past me, driving too fast. I hold the phone to my ear as I walk, hoping not to be connected while the traffic is so loud. My body shivers through another cramp and I stop and press my hand to my tummy. I am now third in the queue.

I stand still on the kerb, and the music has become a little hypnotic. It's all chorus, the kind of repetitive sound that might make a prisoner confess to things they hadn't done. There's no one singing the lyrics, but I can hear them anyway, because the tune is so familiar. I am now second in the queue, the voice tells me.

But still, I can't help feeling that 'Ain't No Mountain High Enough' is a bad choice for a clinic, because some mountains are too high.

'Haringey Health Centre,' says a female voice, human, this time. 'Are you registered with us?'

'Yes.'

'Surname?'

'Knox.'

'Date of birth please?'

'First of the fourth, nineteen eighty-eight.'

'April Fool's!'

'Yes.'

'This isn't a joke?'

She sounds angry now.

'No.'

My birth date is a joke that I have been aware of for many years.

'And what's the address?'

'Eighteen Warwick Road.'

'Middle initial?'

'June,' and then I realise that isn't an initial.

'And you're Lois?'

'Yes.'

'Well done,' she says, which makes me feel oddly proud. 'How can I help?'

'I'd like to make an appointment,' I say.

There's a short silence.

'How's next Wednesday?'

'I was hoping for today . . .'

'We can only do that for emergencies. Is it an emergency?'

'I'm not sure.'

'What's the nature of your condition?'

'I've just had a miscarriage in a toilet.'

'Oh dear,' the woman says. 'Is the bleeding heavy and continuous?'

'No. It's mostly stopped.'

'Let me see what we can do.'

Her tone is a little blank, like she's a shop assistant telling someone they don't have a chosen shoe in the right size. She must hear about lots of conditions.

'Can you do twelve forty-five?'

That's three hours to cover a ten-minute walk.

'Yes,' I tell her.

'Just make sure to call if you're not coming,' she says. 'After three missed appointments we have to de-register you.'

And then she hangs up.

2

DYLAN

'Do you want a 5p bag?'

I don't think so. I have a pack of frozen peas and a cottage pie on the conveyor and both my hands work. I also saw a turtle on Facebook recently that had its flipper caught in a carrier.

'I'm OK, thanks.'

But then, these things are frozen. They'll be cold in my hand, and even if I put them in my pocket, the heat will make them melt. I should've brought a bag with me. These are basic life skills.

She scans the items and I tap my card and hold my breath. Noah's rolling over a little tube of sweets next to the till. He's doing it just enough to scruff up the paper that goes around the outside, without getting it out of the rack. It's making this squeaky, scratchy noise, and even though he's not asking for it, he's staring up at me hopefully. I should stop him because he's damaging it, but it's keeping him quiet, so I will let this tiny vandalism go. Sorry Asda.

The machine beeps and the payment screen flashes, 'Declined'. The woman at the till looks at me.

'It's been declined,' she says.

I want to tell her I can read. I also want to explain that this is a surprise and not the reason I turned down the carrier bag. I did that for the turtles.

But instead I just shrink a little bit. My shoulders rise up, I feel a hot prickle creep up my neck and my forearms itch.

There are two people behind us: a little old lady and a fat guy who looks like he doesn't see much light. The fat guy sighs and I can feel my face flush red and I hope he doesn't notice. He's got a basket full of junk: crisps, chocolates, lager, salami. Nothing that requires any more than opening a packet.

'Have you got another card?'

The cashier is expressionless. She has gold-rimmed glasses with oblong lenses and her hair is pulled tight in a grey-black bun.

I don't have another card. I have exactly what's on this one until tomorrow.

'Can you take the peas off, please?'

She starts doing it and there's still no expression from her, but the fat guy – who has quite a sweaty face – puts his hand on the paused conveyor belt and shifts his weight. He crosses one foot in front of the other like his chauffeur's late, when actually he just wants to guzzle Jammie Dodgers on his way home to slutfest.com.

The till woman nods at me and I tap, and again it says, 'Declined'. Noah's still fiddling with the sweets. The hot prickles rush right across my chest and I want to scratch my arms, but I'm wearing long sleeves and a cardigan and I can't get at the skin. Maybe I could huff about the reader being broken and pretend to go to the cashpoint. But there's almost no food at the flat and the corner shop costs more and I don't know what to do. I'm holding the card in the air, but it's empty, just a little bit of useless plastic. I might as well be waving a toy wand.

I put it down on the counter and reach into my pocket, but my jeans are too tight. I wrestle out my keys, and with them comes fluff, and then I go back in and can feel the hard edges of a 50p. I reach a bit further and there's a 20p, the dotted ridges of a 10p, and I can barely get my fingers around them because the pocket is so small. As I pull them out, I pray they don't go flinging across the floor. The pie is £1.49, but the peas are 79p. I look at the woman and speak really quietly, like I can whisper in a voice that only she can hear.

'Can you put the peas back on and take the pie off?'

But as I give her the coins, it sounds more like the words are stuck at the top of my throat and I'm a pathetic little girl.

I try to give the woman a look that says 'sorry', without having to say it. I would apologise, but the fat guy's right there, so I'm not saying sorry to anyone. She's not saying anything either, just doing what I've asked, and I don't know if that's to stop me feeling bad or just that she's seen this so much before. She picks the pie up and puts it on a little pile of other people's things that never made it through: light bulbs, J-cloths, a bag of spuds. I should've just gone for baked potatoes. Ready meals are a massive waste of money. She taps her till to take the pie off, but something goes wrong and she gives a little sigh and taps some more buttons.

Someone else has joined the queue – another bloke – and the fat guy turns around and rolls his eyes at him, just to make it clear that he's not the one slowing everyone down from whatever very important things they're in Asda to do.

Something rushes up in me, turning my blood hot, and I stare right at his fat, sweaty face and say to him, 'Don't worry, you'll get your biscuits soon.'

And he's got nothing to say. Nothing. Because he knows, really, that he spends his days eating biscuits and wanking.

He's a biscuit wanker. I'm wondering if I should tell him this, but then the machine beeps and the till opens and she drops in my coins and hands me back a penny.

'Would you like the receipt?' asks the cashier.

'Yes, please,' I say, because if I walk out with a bag of frozen peas, then security will think I've nicked them.

I shove the peas in my coat pocket, take Noah by the hand and we head towards the exit. I exhale and feel the skin on my face begin to cool as we walk through the shop. I take a deep breath and the supermarket smells like the inside of a huge cardboard box, but with these massive vents pushing around dirty air.

When I was a kid, I loved how supermarkets smelled of bread, even the bits without bread in them. And then Dad told me it was a scam: the bread smell was fake and they used it to make you hungry and that's how they get you. He died when I was thirteen, and these life lessons are my inheritance.

As we get to the door, Noah yanks at my arm and points to a massive plastic gnome in a tux.

'Wow. Mummy, look!'

'Oh, yes.'

'What do you think it's for?'

'Well, I think it's just for looking at, Noh.'

'No, it's a toy. You can play with it.'

'We don't need any gnomes, Noh.'

The gnome comes up to my knee and costs thirty quid.

I walk out of the supermarket and a woman clips my elbow as she passes and I nearly trip over Noah and take him with me. She ploughs on, glued to her phone, not worried about who she leaves in her wake. She's got this giant yellow mac on, so the world can see her but she doesn't have to look at anyone. It makes her look like a massive toddler.

'Are you OK, Mummy?'

'Yes, Noah.'

'Why did that woman push you, Mummy?'

'Because she's rude, Noah. Some people are like that.'

She doesn't even look back. I wonder why she didn't do an online food shop, a woman like her. I wonder when she last had sex. If her bush is unkempt or bald as a plumber's head.

We step out into the car park and the sound of the North Circular fills the air. It's a constant whisper, like when you hold a shell to your ear, but instead of hearing the sea, you hear a dual carriageway.

'Are we going to the playground?'

He's staring straight up at me with his deep blue eyes, his thick brown fringe just creeping past his brows. His mouth is open, pleading like a chick after some worms.

'Yes, but just five minutes.'

We cross between parked cars to the sun-bleached playground in the corner. It's penned in with a big red wall and over the other side is the road and the rush of cars gets louder here. This is our morning break. A bit of air for him, a tiny breather from cold calls for me. In the afternoons, I take him to the park near the school he'll be joining next week, because he needs airing twice a day, like a puppy.

He scrambles up the climbing frame, beaming down at me before waving his arms in the air and pretending to fall. He does it every time and even though he's joking, my heart thuds as I smile back and waggle my finger at him.

He'll be the funny kid, I reckon. The one who lifts a room.

His smile fills my heart, but it also makes him look just like JD and sometimes that makes me shiver.

Like JD's in my boy, staring out: a perfect little stamp of him,

to be with me forever. A smile that always meant something
bad.

Where you been, Dilly?

But Noah's smile is good. It means he is climbing and free and
needs no one to help him conquer his world, just his own two
hands and feet. And Noah will never have to see his dad's smile,
of course, because Noah believes his dad died before he was
born.

So, get up there, Noh.

I exhale and sit back and watch, put my hands on my belly,
rest them over my C-section scar. Noah's four now, but ever
since he was born and those first days after being stitched
up, my fingers stray to that line. A little reminder that he will
always be mine. One good, big scar to make up for all the little
bad ones.

I breathe and watch Noah play. I pull out my phone, tap
through to my blog, 'One Day Soon'. Every time I look at it, I
feel like some needy American teen from the noughties: 'Hey
guys, check my blog! Tadd smiled at me in the cafeteria! Should
I try bangs?'

But it's anonymous, and a place to put my thoughts before
they evaporate like farts in the night. The views counter hasn't
moved.

So I cycle through my apps: email, news, Instagram, a quick
spin of each to say hello, like they're old pals.

My email inbox is empty because no one wants my book;
there's been a flood in Bangladesh; a man with one leg has had
his benefits stopped; @Miss_bakealot is piping 'You are enough'
on a Black Forest gateau.

I dunno if I am, to be honest.

I holler over to Noah.

'Noh, three more minutes, OK?'

His face sinks a bit, but he nods. When we get home, I'll work and he will play. Then I'll make soup for lunch. There are onions that I can caramelise. There is some veg stock that can go in after, then the peas and some pepper. Simmer, blend and serve with a bit of bread.

Tomorrow I get paid.

3

LO

I walk along the main road to Asda as a bus judders past and my phone is still in my hand like a comforter. The air is chilly, but the sun has dissolved any clouds, and light pings off wing mirrors and shop windows. These few hours while Scout is at nursery are meant to be for writing posts, client feedback, wading through emails. But it's hard to focus when I can feel myself bleeding into cheap tissue. I walk through the first set of automatic doors into the supermarket.

A collection of gnomes stand at the entrance; they're dressed in wedding garb and they're thirty quid each. I take a photo to use later in the week if I'm running short on content. Maybe with a poll: 'Should I buy this gnome? YES/ALSO YES.'

I feel a warm wetness seeping into my leggings and as I head into the supermarket I clip someone walking the other way with my elbow. She passes by before I can apologise and so I continue towards the aisle with the sanitary products, going the long way around to save facing the rows of nappies and smiling baby faces.

I can already hear the well-intentioned support I'll receive from my mum: 'at least you have a daughter', 'at least you can

27

get pregnant'. Nothing helpful starts with 'at least'.

As if having one leg means you aren't allowed to mourn losing the other.

I find a pack of twenty heavy-duty post-partum pads and pull them off the shelf, but I am not post-partum. I have nothing to show for the pregnancy hormones in my veins. But I need the pads that won't leave me bleeding onto a waiting-room chair like before.

And then I am standing in the fruit aisle, holding a bunch of bananas for Scout's post-nursery snacking. I become aware of the weight in my left hand and the pads tucked under my right arm and realise I don't know how long I've been there. A woman looks at me. She's about my age with her hair back in a low pony. I wonder if she's recognised me because she's about to speak and I don't think I can do this now.

If she says, 'Are you @the__lo__down__?' I'll say yes and we'll smile and neither of us will quite know what to do next. I haven't got a smart line today.

'Sorry, could I just . . .?'

She points to some oranges.

'Oh, yes, of course,' I say, standing back and laughing more than I need to. 'I was lost among the Granny Smiths!'

She just smiles and adds a bag of oranges to her trolley.

Once she's gone, I leave, too, eight Fairtrade bananas in my hand. At least half of them will go off before we eat them, but because they're Fairtrade I feel I should buy more. I don't know what would happen if I bought an unfairly traded banana, but I feel like it would be bad.

I move through the store and pick up another pair of grey school trousers for Scout's first day at Reception, pay and make my way to the disabled toilet. It's far worse than the loo at Little Tykes. There's a long black hair dangling from the hot tap and the mirror is cracked in one corner. The bleach can't hide the smell of stale urine. I balance my phone on top of the empty, soap dispenser, which has dried pink residue beneath it. I cover the bloodied gusset of my pants with a sanitary pad, but I should have bought some new knickers too. I pull my leggings up and get out as quickly as I can.

I have two and a half hours before my appointment, so I head to the store's café and sip from my reusable water bottle. I need stillness. I watch people walk by, consumed by lists of things to do and things to buy, and get my phone out and start scrolling again. I wonder if anyone else is sitting in a supermarket café bleeding and waiting. I don't know who to speak to, so I start to write.

Today I miscarried. I am two hours from going to a clinic to make sure all foetal matter has come away. It will be clinical, it will be purely biological and there will be limited room for the emotional. The physicality of passing an embryo sac is something I have never dwelled on in our first miscarriages. Now that unmistakable feeling is flooding back as I sit here alone in a supermarket café. I wasn't even aware I was pregnant and so maybe I shouldn't mourn something I didn't even know was there. But he or she was there and I am here, grieving the loss of a little part of me #babylossawareness.

I upload the post to Instagram with a blank grey image.

My phone lights up.

4

DYLAN

We get back home and I open the shared front door. On the floor is a pile of post and I flip through it as we go up the stairs to the flat. There's a gas bill, loan statement, pizza flyer. The carpet on the tiny landing is ragged, but our flat is clean. I open the door, put the post on the kitchen counter, then lead Noah to his room and hold my breath because I need him to help now, by making life easy.

'Right, what do you want to play?'

He doesn't reply.

'Hey, Noh, how about Duplo?'

I use my excited voice and open his little box of plastic blocks. Sometimes this part goes badly and he doesn't want to be alone. He shrugs.

'Can you play with me today, Mummy?'

It's a tiny little punch in the heart.

'Noah, you know I have to work, darling.'

He does his disappointed face, but he knew that would be the answer. A mum should play, like they do on the toy ads. Lie on the carpet with neat hair and do educational learning. But you can't do that and earn money. I kiss him on the head.

'OK, Mummy's going to do some work now.'

I watch as he tips the box over onto the floor. He has learned to be a self-contained little boy who makes his toys talk to each other, or have fights, or make each other dinner.

Even when I got free nursery hours, I never got further than the forms, because forms leave a trace.

Where you been, Dilly?

Noah starts to put some pieces together and I tell myself, like I do every day, to be proud that he is independent.

But a little bit of me aches that he's spent so much time playing alone. If we knew loads of other kids, maybe he'd be building giant Lego castles by now, instead of pretending Duplo people are his mates. In a week, he has to start school and I don't know if he'll love every minute or cry every day, because all he's ever had is me.

I step into the bathroom and wee, then flush and wash my hands. We need more soap. The bar is tiny, like something from a doll's house. I look in the mirror above the sink. This is when I take a tiny break between Noah and work and feel a low guilt for locking myself away from him. But I need two minutes and the bog is my spa.

I look gaunt, flushed. Women of twenty-six should not look this tired. I roll my shoulders back, stick my chest out, but there's no denying I've got tits like a field mouse.

Nothing there, Dilly. It's like shagging a schoolboy.

Black dye is showing at the base of the blonde. The roots are long now, like it's a style choice and not because I'm skint. And the hair dye is hypocrisy. I won't buy carrier bags because they might hurt turtles, but I will happily get the cheapest peroxide, which pisses ammonia into the lakes and seas.

Somewhere under there is my real hair, thin and straight and brownish blonde. Beige, basically. I've got a beige barnet. It looks mousy, and I don't want to look like a mouse, so I dye it when I've got the cash, because I am not ready to fade away just yet.

When I met JD, I was seventeen and had orange hair and he said I looked like the girl from a film called *The Fifth Element*. That was the nice time, at the beginning. I dyed it pink for a bit, then blue, but he didn't like that.

Looks like you wanna fuck a crusty.

I suck in air, breathe out. It'll take more than hair dye to sort this, let's be honest. Men don't want single mums and their burdens, and they don't want women with scars on their arms, little marks of their troubled teens. Or if they do, they think they can just say nice things to you until a shag falls out, like chucking coins in a fruit machine.

Now get to work, Dyl, you've had your me time.

My laptop and headset are on the kitchen counter and cover half of it. This is my 'office'. When they chopped this little terrace into two flats, they didn't consider the home-working revolution. Or that humans might live in them. Noah used to do these massive jumps from the sofa to the rug that made the whole place shudder and I had to make him stop because of the noise for Mrs Younis downstairs. She never complains, because she's old and polite, but she looks one loud bang away from a heart attack.

I use an 89p 'reporter's notepad' to mark the edge of the

workspace and the beginning of the kitchen. I could work at our little dining table by the bay window, but that is a social space. It is where we eat together. It is six paces away and important to separate work from life.

From where I stand to make my calls, I can reach the kettle, the mugs, the tap and the fridge. I stand when I'm working because it helps give your voice energy, and I work on commission.

But I'm good at it, so it's fine. I don't have the option to not be.

I lease water coolers and coffee machines for a company called H2-Oh, and last week I completed five twelve-month deals. Five sales is a great week, and my line manager emailed to say, 'Excellent effort, Dylan!'

I picture the people I'm talking to, just to keep my mind active. Yesterday, an old guy called Greg Dawlish had 'absolutely zero interest in water coolers or continuing this call', and I imagined him at a Henry VIII banquet, served on a silver platter with an apple in his mouth and a maid pulling off his arm to chew it like a goose leg. When you picture a man like that, he can say what he wants and it doesn't matter.

I put on my headphones and open up ChatTeam. The screen is familiar: its grey-and-blue logo, the little username box with flashing cursor just waiting to suck in your password. While it all loads, I open the envelopes on the counter. The gas bill is the usual. Consolidated Finance Services wish to inform me that my introductory offer has now expired and I will revert to their standard APR of 27.9% for the next eighty-four easy monthly payments. Thanks for the update.

My phone buzzes with a new text. A message from Mum. She wonders if I've got time for a call next week.

Maybe. We haven't spoken for months and she hasn't seen

Noah since his second birthday. But then those calls sit with me for months afterwards, so maybe not.

On the headset, I hear the purr of a phone. A female voice.

'Kensons.'

I widen my eyes, take a deep breath and begin my day of selling water to people who already have taps.

'Oh hello there! I wonder if you could help. I'd really love to speak to the office manager. Might that be you?'

And as I speak, I throw out my biggest smile.

5

LO

The oven clock glares '20:28'. Scout is asleep upstairs and I'm at the kitchen table, which is also my office. Glitter winks at me from knots in the wood, memories of past crafting projects. Johno is still not home, so it's just me with 33,728 well-meaning strangers. After this morning's miscarriage post, 1,000 more followers came to support me.

The doctor said to 'just' wait and rest. Like it's a graze that will heal. I was five weeks pregnant, so it's much like a heavy period. Almost nothing. Just pop a few more ibuprofen.

I flick my thumb over the screen of my phone and wait for it to refresh.

Dozens of people believe I am brave.

Hundreds are thinking of me.

Many understand what I'm going through.

I wonder if Amara has seen it. But you can't just WhatsApp, 'Sorry, love', and she has baby Theo, who is probably sucking the life out of her right now.

I lean back and rest a hand on my bloated stomach and wonder if it was a boy or a girl. I wonder at what point those cells become someone. When they grow a penis or build a vagina. When they decide if he is going to be creative or if she's got a mathematical mind. Whether he had my eyes or she had Johno's.

I stare at the geometric floor tiles, a design decision I fought Johno for and now regret every time I look down. There's an abandoned chip by the table leg, but I don't have the energy to pick it up. I keep scrolling. A woman in Utah tells me she had a stillborn baby girl at thirty-two weeks. They don't know how they'll pay the hospital bills, but she must take faith in her husband's love and the knowledge that this is God's plan and she will pray that I too can see that one day soon.

Several people believe I am helping others by shining a light on the unspoken shame of losing a baby. But I don't think I was shining a light. I just needed to feel I wasn't alone.

A woman on the south coast wants to tell me she has had her rainbow baby after seven miscarriages, and that however low I feel now, there will always be hope and a new day. Rainbow babies are the ones that come after miscarriage. After heavy clouds, there's a rainbow. After seven deaths, there's a birth. Mother Nature's cruellest game of snakes and ladders.

Another woman says she hopes people will respect my privacy at this time, even though I posted publicly.

A woman in Manchester thinks she may be miscarrying now and she can't tell her family because she's not supposed to be pregnant. I message and tell her to please call a doctor. She tells me she can't, because the doctor will tell her parents. And then I can see that she's not a woman at all, but she's fifteen or sixteen. So I tell her that hospitals have to respect her privacy and can't speak to her parents without permission, though I'm not sure if that's true. But I am sure that if she's pregnant and bleeding she needs to see someone.

People send tear-faced emojis and kisses.

Amara wants to meet and give me a hug.

I need to tell Mum, but can't face hearing 'at least you . . .'

Johno has called twice and messaged eight times.

This was no way for him to find out. I have been unkind. He started messaging at lunchtime, and I could picture him, pre-packed sandwich in hand, sat on a wooden bench in that grey plaza, flicking about on his phone: football videos, girls in bikinis, wife having miscarriage.

I just couldn't call him and hear the silence again, so I turned to strangers on the internet.

The door opens and he crashes in, the letter box clanking. If he's any louder, he'll wake Scout. He looks wild-eyed and he's holding pink tulips and all I can think of is the colour of the water and it just makes me want to be away from him. He walks round the table towards me, flowers aloft like it's my birthday. I start walking around the other side like he's a ghost and I'm Pac-Man.

'Lo . . .'

'We're not celebrating. Flowers are for celebrating.'

I feel like my whole body has contracted, my shoulder blades tighten, my lungs compress. Then it floods out of me like a dam bursting, my phone shakes in my hand and my shoulders surge up and down and he wraps himself around me. I'm just there in his arms and he's warm and smells of the day. He smells of the Tube and coffee and the tang of dried sweat. He smells of him and he's a blanket around me, so we stay like that for a while. My arms are almost bound together by his hug and the blue glow of my phone is pressed against his chest. It lasts a minute or ten, I'm not really sure, and then he speaks.

'You didn't answer my calls.'

'I couldn't tell you over the phone. I just wanted to see you.'

'I found out on Instagram.'

He stands back so we can see each other, but I can't look at him. He speaks quietly.

'Lo, I found out on Instagram.'

'I know! I know it's shit! I just wanted to tell people. To help them. To help me.'

His brown eyes look pained. The same eyes that lit up as we exchanged vows and clouded over when he lost his dad. Eyes that don't look at me as they once did.

'I'm sorry,' I say.

I want him to ask me how I feel, even if I can't answer. I want him to ask if the pain is manageable, even if it reminds me of what we've lost. I want him to cry at the loss of a hotchpotch of cells that might have had the same chestnut eyes as him and Scout. But he keeps looking intently at me and we stand in silence.

'Why didn't you come home earlier?'

'It was the worst day.'

I stare up at him.

'Sorry, I mean it was just busy.'

He is an accountant at a music label, but he knows that quarterly finance reports are not as traumatic as a life inside you being flushed down the toilet, so I don't say it.

'I'm so sorry,' he says, and he pulls me in again and kisses the top of my head. 'Can we just lie down, maybe? It's all . . . a lot.'

Yes. It is 'a lot'. And it's more when you are silent. Like a little protective shell closes around your heart, and I just want to know if it's because your words hurt too much to say or because you just don't want to hear mine, and that's why I couldn't call.

So we walk through to the living room and the green velvet sofa. It isn't big enough for two adults to lie side by side, so he throws off the back cushions to give us more room. He does this carefully, piles them neatly, a way to show this is serious. This is not the casual heaping of cushions that might happen before watching a quick sitcom episode, but something more deliberate. Like an invalid is here who shouldn't see sudden movements. We lie down and fit tightly, me in his arms again like a bug in its cocoon. I've stopped crying and we just lie there, breathing.

He wishes I hadn't announced it to the world before I told him and he's right. That will be sitting in him somewhere. He probably wishes I hadn't told the world at all. But I told the world because when I tell him, he no longer knows what to say.

'I'm sorry I didn't speak to you first.'

'It's OK.'

'I just felt overwhelmed and needed to say something.'

'I understand.'

With the first one we lost, he came running across town. I sent a text to say I was bleeding, and he walked straight out of a meeting and was there thirty minutes later with a cab to take me to hospital.

By that night, I was on a ward, with the curtains drawn around our bed, and he was dozing in an armchair by my side with our coats for a blanket. We were waiting for an eight-week-old amniotic sac to pass, which I could have done at home, but they wanted to observe, given how much blood I'd lost. In the night, a nurse came to change my pad and by lamplight she tipped the contents into a cardboard kidney dish.

'It looks like everything has passed now,' she said.

Then Johno was by my side asking to see it. She sort of paused, not sure if he should, and while she thought about it, he leaned over and looked, so I did, too. It was a little purple sack in a dark red puddle and a sting hit the back of both of our eyes.

'What do you do with it?' he asked.

'We'll dispose of it carefully.'

And then she took it away and I didn't want to know any more. But he told me, two weeks later, that he couldn't stop thinking about it.

'You can't bury a thing that small or make a cask the size of a matchbox,' he said. 'So it must be incinerated.'

And that thought has stuck with me ever since. We left it there like a forgotten glove and they tossed it on the fire. As if it were an insignificant and replaceable thing. But it wasn't, it was a very specific collection of cells that would have made a very specific person. One with different fingerprints but the same fair hair as Johno, maybe. One that might have had blue eyes like mine. One that might have been a little shorter or taller, a little chattier or quieter. One that might have slept differently or fed differently. One that might have nuzzled into me in their own special way.

In the weeks after that first time, he tried to say reassuring things. 'At least it was early,' as though that made it matter less. Or, 'It'll work out next time,' which was an empty lie.

After the second time, he suggested a therapist, which we couldn't afford, and a memorial tree, which was ridiculous as we lived in a flat.

Maybe the fifth feels more ordinary, and so now he's saying nothing.

But I need some words, even the wrong ones, to show he's lost in the darkness, too.

I lay my palm flat on his chest.

'I'm sorry I didn't call you.'

'It's OK.'

'It's not. I can't imagine finding out like that.'

He shakes his head very gently.

'It's OK. What should we do for you? Did the doctor say? Do you want a hot-water bottle?'

'Maybe later.'

'Maybe some tea? To help the cramps.'

'I've taken painkillers.'

'I'll run you a bath later.'

These are the things he offers when he doesn't know what to do. Like I'm something faulty that needs an adjustment. He squeezes me a little, strokes my hair.

'Johno?'

'Yes.'

'It would help me if I knew how you felt.'

He exhales and it feels heavy. Not a sigh or a huff, but a little gust of resignation.

'Well . . . I feel sad.'

I wait. Give him space to say more, but nothing comes.

'Please, Johno.'

'Well . . .'

He adopts a tone. Like he's explaining something very obvious but trying to do it in his softest, kindest voice. Like he shouldn't have to say any of this, but if he must, he will make it clear and simple and stripped of feeling. It's the voice he uses for Scout when he's reading a bedtime story and doesn't want to excite her with his funny accents: a soft monotone for willing her to sleep.

'I feel sad that another baby's gone, and I wonder who it would have been. I wonder if it would have been a boy or a girl, and if it would be nicer for Scout to have a sister than a brother. Someone to share clothes with, and for me to perfect my plaits on. But also, maybe, a little glad I didn't know we

41

were pregnant, because I've had no time to think about it . . .'

And then his voice cracks: a slip and a sharpening, half a note higher.

'. . . And I feel sad that you couldn't call me. That those strangers had to know first, and I don't know what I've done that means you can't call me. I don't know what I've done wrong before.'

'Johno, you haven't—'

'But mostly I want to know what to do for you.'

My head sits on his chest, my palm on it too, just above my face-down phone, the heat of it warming my hand.

'I just want this, Johno. I want you to tell me. I don't want flowers, I want to know how you feel.'

'Well, that's how.'

We stay silent, and I rub my thumb up the side of the phone, causing the covered screen to glow a little halo against his shirt.

'And what else?'

He begins to speak, pauses. There's more, but he can't share it.

'You can tell me.'

'It might upset you.'

I look up at him.

'I'd rather know.'

His tone shifts again, quieter now, like a doctor delivering bad news.

'I wonder if maybe we can find a positive.'

I don't speak, because I don't understand, and he continues.

'And the only thing is, it'll give us a little more time to save. We've still got no financial cushion, really, since buying the house. And I still wobble a bit when I think about the mortgage.'

'Yes.'

'I'm sorry. But, if you want to know, that's what I'm feeling.'

'I do.'

'That doesn't mean I'm glad we lost it.'

'No.'

'Just that you have to try to find one positive, in the tragedy. Not positive. That's the wrong word.'

'It's OK, Johno, I understand.'

A second baby doesn't quite fit the spreadsheet. Maybe he's relieved, and he doesn't want to say.

'And the whole work situation,' he adds.

'Yes.'

'I mean, Kwame's stopped wearing trainers and started with loafers, which I think might mean he has board aspirations.'

This is how he moves the conversation on. Kwame is his boss, recently promoted, with Johno doing Kwame's old job, without the raise or title. And whenever he wants to placate me, to give me some detail of his life beyond these walls, Johno tells me about Kwame's newest chunky-knit cardigan, or his latest tortoiseshell glasses, or the little tribes in the office, how the interns look like reality-TV contestants, how the A and Rs look like dads from a covers band. And so I play along.

'Do you think it might be time for you to wear some grown-up shoes?'

'Maybe if I get Assistant Finance Director permanently. That's a shoe role.'

He rolls his shoulders a little. I rest my head on his chest again and can hear the soft, faint tap of his heart.

After a while, he stretches up his toes and breaks the silence.

'Can you believe our little girl starts school next week,' he says.

Like that's it.

It's a statement. Not one that needs an answer. Like he's discussing the prospect of rain with a colleague.

Because this is what he needs, of course: to look forward, to move on.

As if nothing ever happened.

6

SEPTEMBER

DYLAN

Noah is immaculate for his first day. I have cut his hair to a perfect fringe and it's so clean there's a little shine across the front like a halo.

His bag does not have the federation logo on it because those ones are twelve quid and since when did kids become billboards? He has a plain, navy school bag, which cost £6 and is listed as acceptable on the school website. He's standing by the door like a miniature soldier and I wanna squeeze him till he pops.

They will not see a poor kid, they will see a perfectly neat one, and bollocks to them, anyway.

'Can I have some milk, Mummy?'

'We've run out, Noh. Is squash OK?'

He nods and I make some. I watch him drink it and when he's done, I finish the rest. I give the counter a last wipe and notice a dried porridge blob on the laminate by the sink and start to pick it off.

When I first saw this flat, I was so happy to find something that didn't have damp or a metal grate over the door that I didn't think about schools, so I am #blessed to be in a good catchment area. Chandling has a massive banner out front telling everyone it's 'Outstanding', like it's a kid showing off a swimming certificate.

But school is a new stage. Another list that Noah's name is on, another database where he could be found.

Where you been, Dilly?

There are 120 kids per year, seven years, plus parents. That's 1,000 people through the gates in fifteen minutes, and anyone could walk in. It's not like there are bouncers.

I'm scrubbing at the porridge and in its place is now a pale patch of scuffed laminate. We need to go. I give Noah a big kiss on the top of his head.

'Come on, Noh-Noh, let's make some new friends!'

It's bright and warm, a little late-summer fightback after a cold spell, and by the time we get to school, it's heaving. Little lines of people streaming in from all the streets around and through the main gate, which is bright red and yellow like a poisonous frog.

You can already see how it works: Converse mums in one gang dressed in 'athleisure'; the mums who shop at the market; the mums who come in their slippers. There's a group of three women standing together who all have eyebrows that look like they've been done with a marker pen.

There are a lot of dads too. Maybe this is normal now, dads at the school gates. Mine only picked me up once, and he stood there with this big grin and a bag of sweets, shouting 'Surprise!' with mum next to him all quiet and it felt like the best day of my life. Took me years to work out he'd just been sacked again.

But today there are dads everywhere, and I thought this

would be a place for women. It's crowded and I'm going a bit face-blind. All these men are about JD's age. They all dress the same, too; like blokes all choose their jeans and trainers when they're fourteen and that'll do them until they die.

I can feel my neck prickle and my chest get tight and I just sort of stop.

'OI!'

'HAHA!'

'Hello!'

'Fancy seeing you here.'

Some kind of panto has broken out next to me. Two mums doing a greeting ritual, with massive grins and swaying back and forth.

'KAMAL. Water bottle!'

'Scooter, please.'

'Oliver, put your shoe back on.'

'Quickly!'

There are shouted conversations all around me. A man jogs past, dragging his boy behind. A kid bumps my leg. A man brushes my back. It's like we're in a wave pool.

There's a tug on my jeans.

'Can I have my water?'

I look down and it's a little girl.

'What?'

She stares up at me, then spins around.

'Maya!'

The girl's mum takes her hand and smiles at me.

'Sorry! So many people! Maya, this way.'

I hold Noah's hand tighter.

'You're not her mummy,' he says.

'No, I know.'

It's like I'm at a foreign train station at rush hour. Everyone

47

else knows their way and I can't find the departures board. There's a clatter of metal on concrete as some woman drops her kid's scooter. My body jerks and I want to swing at her. It's like there's an electric charge running from my belly to my arms and it's making everything twitch.

Everyone's rushing. I never thought there'd be this many blokes.

Noah starts to wriggle his hand out of mine.

'Noah, stop!'

A woman with big red glasses turns round to look at me. Noah looks up.

'Is it over there?'

And he's right, even though he can't read, because it's obvious, and there are four teachers and an A-frame that says: 'RECEPTION. Welcome to our new learners'.

And this is it. I'm just supposed to hand him over. Give him to someone to whisk away to the back of the building.

'Are they new kids too?'

'Yes, Noah.'

'Can you take me there?'

'Yes.'

But I don't move. The playground we're in has a metal fence around it that's about two metres high and any adult with working legs and arms could get over in thirty seconds. Then there's a small fence for what looks like the Reception playground, which is waist-high.

And that's it. No security at a school, just doughy women who know how to do finger painting.

Noah tugs my hand, because he wants to be with the other children. I hear a voice behind me.

'Are you in the queue?'

There's a woman walking a cargo trike with three kids in it.

Three kids in uniform and all their bags loaded into a wooden crate on the front.

'What?'

'Year Two – are you in the Year Two line?'

'No.'

'Do you mind if I squeeze through?'

There are queues growing all over the playground and we're in the middle of one, so I step aside and she begins to unload her little gang.

Noah looks up at me.

'Are we going there, Mummy?'

'Yes.'

People keep coming. You couldn't run now, it's too packed. But I want to leave. I want to take Noah home and close the door and move away before the council realise he's not at school. I feel something in my stomach, like a dryness. It runs from the pit of me to the back of my throat.

'Mummy?'

There's a long line now for Noah's class.

All the teachers have name boards and his one, Ms Carole, looks exactly like I'd expect a Reception teacher to look. She's in her twenties but dressed like she's about to retire and has this big grin that hasn't dropped since we arrived.

'Yes, let's go.'

It feels like I'm walking slowly, or everything around me has speeded up. The kids are all shouting and screaming and there are too many of them. Will they be kind to my boy? Will they let him play their games and sit with him at lunch?

We reach her line and the teacher smiles at me. And even though she's been smiling at everyone, when she looks in your eyes, it's like she's smiling just for you.

'And who do we have here?'

She turns her beam down to my boy.

'He's Noah Rayne.'

She ticks his name off a list on her clipboard, bends down a little further.

'Hello, Noah. Are you excited about your first day?'

He gazes up at her, but he doesn't answer straight away. Maybe he's found this morning overwhelming, too, and wants to come back with me and close the door and never leave again.

'Yes,' he says.

'Well good. We're going to have a fun first day of singing songs and getting to know each other.'

He likes her already.

'Would you like to join your new classmates, Noah?'

She points to the line and he starts to go, but I've still got his hand. He looks up at me like we're all done, but I keep hold of him.

I kneel down and hug him so tight I crumple his uniform. I kiss him on the cheek and hold it there. I hold my lips to his soft skin and press on the cheekbone until he starts to wriggle.

'He'll be fine,' says the teacher, but I'm still looking at Noah.

'Now you be good, and have fun, and you don't go anywhere – not anywhere, Noh – without telling your teacher.'

'Yes, Mummy.'

His hand slips out of mine and into hers, and she leads him two steps to the back of the queue, then turns around and starts to talk over my shoulder: 'And who do we have here?'

And that's it.

I'm handing him over. I stand as he leaves and my stomach rolls forward and my chest empties of air.

It feels like I'm falling. Like I've taken a jump off the high board at a swimming pool and I want to step back. Like I've made a terrible mistake because I don't know how to swim and I just want to grasp the air and stop myself dropping, but it's too late.

There are hundreds of kids and hundreds of adults, but all I can see is Noah. He smiles at the kids behind and in front of him and they smile back and none of them know where to look, so they stare at the ground or their parents or at each other. Just look directly at each other and say nothing.

This is where it begins for him – new friends and learning and stepping away from me.

A bell rings and the teachers begin to lead them in. Noah's class goes second, into the little Reception playground and on into their room. The teacher opens the door and points the way, and through the window I can just see the top of his head bobbing by, the rest of him obscured by posters Blu-Tacked to the glass.

They all file in and the teacher follows.

She doesn't lock the door.

Any kid could walk out and any adult could walk in.

This could be the moment that replays forever. There's my life before today and my life after today: why did you let your son go to school that morning, Ms Rayne?

My head feels light.

I breathe in through my nose, out through my mouth.

My chest's folding in.

I breathe deeper, but there are little spots round my eyes.

And then I feel the bang right in my chest and it's JD.

He's found us.

Found the school.

Found our boy and me and won't let us go again.

A scream gets stuck halfway up my neck and I can't speak.

He's here and he's gonna take me away and I'm going to throw up on the playground floor.

But it's not JD. It's that woman in her yellow mac, marching through me like I don't exist. Again!

'Sorry,' she says, 'I didn't see you there.'

And then she just moves on, staring at her phone, her thumb skipping about the screen. That's twice now, and I know exactly who she is – she'll be in a rush to catch up with her mates over an almond-milk latte. She'll tell them she uses a moon cup but actually stuffs her fanny with Tampax.

They're all about the sisterhood those lot, until you need real help.

7
LO

Scout is in her uniform, but as we stand by the door I can't quite bring myself to open it. She looks different, like someone else's child, and her blazer swamps her tiny shoulders.

'Ready?'

She looks a little unsure.

'I haven't said goodbye to Daddy.'

But Johno is right there, jogging down the stairs to catch us before we go. He plants a smacker on her fringe, kneels down and looks her in the eye.

'How you feeling?'

'Good.'

'Super-duper good?'

'Super-duper good.'

'Strong?'

He does a little growl and curls up both his biceps.

'Strong,' she says, and he gives her a look.

So she copies his stance, her little sapling arms curled, and gives a throaty growl. Then he gives me a peck and smiles. I feel warmth bridge the gap between us. Johno always knows what to say to Scout. He turns to me.

'And how are you feeling?'

'Good.'

And it's true, because this is the first day I've been able to think about anything other than flushing a little life away.

'Ready for today's content opportunity?' he asks.

He smiles, because this is a joke, but it's also a dig. He describes what I do to his mates as 'a side hustle'. Like I'm filling time between luncheon with the ladies and afternoon bridge club, but always overlooking the money I earn. I'm getting ten grand for the Etisk partnership.

'Always.'

I give him a flat smile and turn to Scout.

'Come on, little nugget, let's fly!'

She smiles back at me and I feel ready and walk out of the door. I'm wearing black leggings and a grey marl jumper that makes me look like a tired extra from *Footloose* and wrap myself in my big yellow mac. I want to look approachable without anyone approaching.

Chandling is five minutes away, Ofsted outstanding, and the reason we live here. About six months after Scout was born, Johno began looking. It was like a military campaign, and he approached it with an accountant's zeal for spreadsheets. He fed in a list of state primary schools in Tube zones one to four that were rated outstanding.

He then took the postcodes for those schools and matched them with Met Police statistics and crossed off those in areas where the crime rate was higher than the London average.

Then he cross-matched this with Rightmove data on areas where the average price of two- or three-bed houses was within our budget. He then added outstanding state secondaries and grammars (mixed or all-girls), because 'it can't hurt' to consider where a six-month-old might do her GCSEs.

By now the list was quite small, and he added his own notes to places he knew. Anything too close to his mum in Watford moved to the bottom of the list. He applied a pale green tinge to those areas that had decent pubs and places to eat. He presented this list to me like a kid showing off artwork.

'It's a bit much,' he said. 'Now's probably the time to admit I twice played Dungeons and Dragons at school.'

So we found a three-bed terraced house, got a crippling mortgage and now, somehow, it's Scout's first day and I'm gripping her hand as we walk down the street. This morning I gave her Honey Cheerios as a breakfast treat and I must have kissed the top of her head twenty times.

As we get closer to the gates, the narrow streets start to fill with stressed parents dragging their children along, shouting at them to hurry. One boy weaves through the throng on a bright red scooter. I used to see this on my way to drop Scout at nursery, and now that we're part of it I wonder how we'll fit.

As we walk in, there are nervous smiles and tiny kisses and the handing over of water bottles. No one smiles at me or looks me in the eye, which is fine because we don't know each other. At least, I don't know them. Some of my followers have told me they live in Haringey too.

I watch the kids pinball around the playground and find myself giving a commentary to Scout.

'Look, Scout, there's a bike shed!'

I tell her this to make her feel comfortable. To make everything new and wonderful and exciting.

'Yeah.'

'Maybe, if you get a bike for Christmas, you'll be able to ride in.'

'Yeah.'

'And this must be where you have playtime.'

'Yeah, I know.'

She's trying to sound blasé to reassure me.

'I wonder what you'll have for lunch? I used to love school puddings.'

'Are they nice?'

'Once, we had chocolate sponge and mint custard.'

'Oh.'

She weighs this up, like it's not surprising and might be acceptable.

'You know what, Scout?'

'What?'

'I'm a bit jealous.'

'Why?'

She gives me one of her sceptical looks.

'You're about to make a whole class of new friends. How exciting is that?'

'Yeah.'

She can tell, I think, that I'm pepping her up.

I squeeze her hand reassuringly, although I'm wondering who really needs reassurance. I keep thinking of the moment I have to turn around and leave her with strangers who might make her feel things that I can't make better because I'm not there.

She looks up at me with a smile of serene indifference and it's Johno's face. It's like his features have been etched onto our little girl. Same deep brown eyes and frown, same dark blonde hair. It's almost cartoonish how much she looks like him and everyone made the same comments when they saw her as a baby:

'Well aren't you Daddy's girl!'

'No need for a DNA test there!'

Even Mum whispered in my ear, 'Don't worry, it's just nature's way of making sure the father sticks around while you're feeling frumpy.'

I carried Scout for nine months, hatched her and nourished her and gave her my body, but he got to leave the genetic stamp.

I put her book bag over her shoulder. It holds seven different pens and a fluffy puppy keyring.

There's a woman wearing a dressing gown next to us, her pink Hello Kitty pyjamas stuffed into Ugg boots. Another woman is in an emerald sari with diamanté kitten heels, like she's about to take to the wedding floor. There's a group of women to my left who are decked in slogan jumpers like a wearied girl band. One reads 'Mother' in a bold font.

My heart pounds and I don't want to let Scout go. I want to wrap her in a hug and take her home for a day of eating Haribos and watching films with a duvet over us. I want to do this while it still might sound like the best day of her life.

She is a tiny woman with feelings and opinions and a sense of humour and I want her to be mine alone. She is a little girl who blows out her cheeks to do impressions of puffer fish whenever she's bored. She fits in my arms so perfectly now, but sometime soon she'll be desperate to escape them and this is where it begins. This is where she starts to learn to live without me. First she needed me to breathe, then she needed me to eat, then to walk and now she needs me to let her go. My heart aches, but I smile, cheeks forced full of positivity.

In the corner of the playground are four teachers, each wearing a white sticker with their name and class handwritten in neat lettering. Ms Carole has a beaming smile that lights her entire face and she looks like a twenty-five-year-old Mrs Tiggy-Winkle.

'Look, Scout, it's your teacher!'

Scout looks over and her face is blank, then awed, then a little afraid, and finally I can see some of what she's thinking.

'Shall we go and say hello?'

I smile from twenty yards away and Ms Carole smiles back, then looks down at Scout as we approach.

'And who do we have here?'

Her voice is very soft and lilting and something you could listen to all day. I wait for Scout to answer.

'I'm Scout.'

'And are you excited about your first day?'

'Yes.'

She delivers this as a statement of absolute certainty. I am Scout, and I'm ready for the world.

'Well, I'm excited, too,' says Ms Carole. 'Now, the first thing we must learn is how to line up for class. Could you join your new classmates?'

She points to a queue of twenty kids, all looking around at their new world. Scout looks at me, and behind those eyes of Johno's is just a flicker of doubt. I kneel down to wrap her in my arms, then clamp a hand on each of her cheeks to give her a massive kiss on the lips.

'Now, you have the best day, OK?'

All I really want to do is cry, or run away with her, but she smiles and nods, says, 'I love you.'

'Now, say bye-bye to Mummy,' says Ms Carole.

And she does. She says, 'Bye, Mummy,' and turns around and walks off to her line as Ms Carole begins the process all over again with a girl clinging to her mother's leg.

'And who do we have here?'

Scout looks back, and I wave and stand my ground, until eventually there is a bell and the little gaggle of wide-eyed infants shuffles forward.

My only child has begun school. Until she has a sibling – if she ever has a sibling – every first for Scout will also be the last time for me. Maybe I'll never get to hear another child of mine say first words, or take first steps, or walk off for a first day at school. Her little, warm hand is like an anchor to me and without it I'm adrift.

I can feel the tears pushing against my eyelids, so I turn on my heel and flick to my phone.

Instagram has fifty-six DMs, forty-two comments, 112 likes.

My inbox has fifty-seven unread emails.

WhatsApp shows twenty-eight new messages.

Jenn, my manager, needs Instagram insights for the recent Etisk ad. She needs these by 9.00 a.m. latest, as the client is chasing.

A woman has sent me a photo of herself expressing in a work-toilet cubicle. She has said if I care about changing the narrative I should share her photo with an @ tag.

Another woman asks if I felt suicidal after my miscarriage.

Amara has texted: *'So sorry to hear about the shit you've gone through, my love. I just want to see you, to hug you and get mascara stains on my shoulder. For now, here's summat to cheer you up . . . Influenza. It's a new one of those gossip sites. It's tiny, but it's mad, and it's all about people like you. I'm addicted. Get yerself over there X.'*

As I read and walk, I feel a jolt as I walk directly into another mum.

'Oh, God, sorry,' I say, 'I didn't see you there.'

She looks at me like I just spat in her face.

8
DYLAN

There were a thousand people here five minutes ago, now it's like the place has been flushed. Some of the parents literally ran away. That woman from the supermarket didn't even look back.

A couple of mums are chatting, toddlers hanging off them, but I'm the only other one left. I just watch Noah's classroom, even though I can't see him and I need to get to work. Every call is an opportunity, they tell us.

'Sorry, we need to lock up now.'

There's a young guy jangling some keys and he gives me a smile. He's just wearing jeans and a polo shirt that shows off his arms.

'First day's always tough, I think. Same every year. Don't worry, kids all love it after a week.'

I smile back but don't say anything and he nods towards the gate. He's the school centurion. Maybe he could stop someone getting in. I smile again, and we look at each other, but now it's time to go.

I start to walk home, do some slow, steady breathing on the way. JD is not here, because he doesn't know where we are.

It's fine, Dyl.

I reach for my phone and scroll a little as I walk.

The ice caps are melting faster than we thought; the Minister of Defence is friends with someone who sells helicopters; no one wants my book; @Mumdamentalist found the first day of school exciting; and the One Day Soon view counter hasn't moved. Maybe it's broken.

My phone screen is smudged, so I rub it on my cardigan.

JD bought me my first smartphone. Just handed it over in the pub, all shiny and new, but no box and him taking care of the bill.

And then he called and messaged whenever we were apart.

Last night was amazing.
I can't stop thinking about you.
What are you doing right now?

It gave me little flutters: a man cared and was only thinking of me.

I flip to Instagram again and it's full of back-to-school pictures and 'First day!' and jokes about drinking Prosecco at the school gates. There is a trend for pretending that you hate your kids, or that cooking for them is too difficult and you'd rather be sucking gin. But it mostly seems to come from Instamums in nice houses with well-behaved husbands and maybe they don't think their kid might be taken away from them.

Or maybe they're all secretly sad to say goodbye and this is how they make themselves feel better about it. Or maybe they all feel weird being in a school again, and it reminds them of being younger.

The last time I was in a school playground, I was sixteen, collecting my GCSE results and heading to the park to get pissed on pocket money. When I got home, Mum wasn't even mad, because an English Lit A among the Ds convinced her I was a child genius. She even gave me some of her wine.

But I just wanted out by then. Away from her and her replacement men. I loved her – she's still my blood – but after Dad died, I loved her less. It's hard to love a woman that moves on that fast.

And after that day, I never went to school again.

So maybe Noah can make up for it.

He can be an A-star kid. Work hard and be nice to his mum and do all the things I couldn't.

Until then, I'll do the work for both of us.

I get to our shared front door just as Mrs Younis comes out.

'Hello, dear!'

She beams when she has something to say. She is tiny and a little hunched over, but when she wants to tell you something, her eyes dance.

'First day today!'

'Yes.'

'Is he a happy boy?'

'Yes, he ran in.'

'And are you a happy mother?'

'Well, it's a bit hard.'

I give her a smile. She has two grown-up boys, and when she sees Noah, her face glows.

'Well, they go away very soon,' she says.

'It feels like it.'

Mrs Younis is lonely, I think. A few months ago, she gave me a key to hers, 'just in case', and I had visions of her keeled over in front of *The One Show*. She looked right into me as she handed it over, like we're all that each other have, and I should give her something back.

So, a week later, I gave her the spare to mine. It felt like she needed it: just a little connection, just to show I trusted her too. And an emergency locksmith costs £300, of course, and I don't have £300.

That's the thing about doing it alone. You lose something and it's gone, there's no one with a backup. If I lost my key, we'd be living in the park. So I asked her to put it somewhere safe, where no one could see it, and she showed me her spot: under a blue ceramic cat on her mantelpiece. The cat is hollow, with a little hole at the bottom. She looked proud, like she was being clever and helpful, and I smiled and immediately regretted giving a stranger a key to our home.

I wanted to pop round for tea and slip it back in my bag while she put the kettle on, but every time I saw her, all that was there was loneliness.

'And how are your boys?'

'Good, good. But boys don't call. If I had a daughter, she would call.'

She looks at me like her sons have been lost at sea. I smile and she smiles back, like this will be my fate too.

'OK,' she says.

'Have a great day.'

I sound like I work at Disneyland.

She heads out and I go up to the flat. I boil the kettle, turn on the laptop and hold my breath. The machine is older than Noah and has more tantrums, bought on tick second-hand, and sometimes it just freezes: locks up like it's having a spasm and nothing happens. But today it's OK. I put milk and one sugar in my tea and take a sip.

I log in to ChatTeam and open my emails. There's one from school, 'A Welcome to Parents'. It has a PDF with three pages of dense text.

Jeez. Three years of teacher training and they've never seen a bullet point.

That can wait until later, because I have a little ritual while I'm working. We're supposed to get through fifty contact calls a day, but when there are little pauses as ChatTeam hits dead phone lines or engaged tones, I email book publishers. This way, it feels like I'm getting paid to be a writer.

There are 847 publishers in the UK, and I have emailed 612. I'm up to the letter R. For each one, I find an email address, or guess at one – info@, admin@, office@ – paste in my message and attach one document.

The_Women_Who_Watch_On.doc.

Dear Sir or Madam,
For your consideration: a novel, *The Women Who Watch On*.
Yours truly,

Dylan Rayne

I keep it simple, so they'll read it, but no one really replies, you just get autoresponses. My last actual message was from a guy that said, 'Sorry, we do gardening books.'

It's a lame thing to do, but I do it like a little game. A thing for me, in those seconds between calls. It took me two years and I wrote most of it on pen and paper and kept it hidden under the mattress because JD wouldn't have liked it.

It's about a woman called Elaine who has an abusive partner. He meets her when she's very low and shows her something that looks like love, but then very slowly he erodes her. He chips away at her mind and her spirit until she feels entirely worthless and he controls her completely.

He never leaves a bruise, but he cuts her off from her family and friends, takes her money, monitors her phone, locks her in their flat.

It has a happy ending though.

Because one day she stabs him right in the heart.

9
LO

It's Friday night and I swirl a chocolate-sauce heart over Scout's ice cream and her eyes sparkle as she grins 'more please'. I'd give her the whole bottle with a straw if it meant she looked at me like that forever. Ice cream drips down her chin from her perfect rosebud lips and I wipe it and pop my finger in her mouth so she doesn't miss a drop.

This has been a big two weeks for her. She's gone from a sandpit and ABCs to a desk and phonics, so today she gets fish fingers, chips and beans, followed by ice cream.

I take a photo of Scout eating, maybe one to print and send to Mum and Dad. My parents don't really understand my world. They frown and prod their phones like they might detonate, and they're yet to download Instagram.

I haven't told Mum about the latest miscarriage because she's from a time when trauma was swept under the recently Hoovered rug, and there was always a worry about what the neighbours would think, while I can't stop thinking about the women who bled alone in peach-and-avocado bathrooms. When I told her about my previous miscarriages, she said, 'What a comfort to already have Scout. You go squeeze that little one tonight.' Like one life makes up for the loss of another.

It's been three weeks since I lost the baby, but the Instagram messages keep coming and I keep posting. Every day at 8.00 p.m., I tell 41,000 women what I'm feeling.

Some of them tell me back. A woman in Kent says I have given her the courage to start trying again. A woman in Australia is worried about me and thinks I need time off.

But I don't have time off, because this is my income, my small oasis of independence. No one in HR can send me an email telling me I'm no longer needed. No one can make me redundant.

In two days I have to post an ad for a new coffee maker and Jenn, my manager, says I need to move the conversation on. She's worried that shifting from miscarriage to macchiatos might jar a little. Jenn is at the social media agency, HMN Hub, and got in touch just before I hit 10,000 followers.

'Your empowering message really chimes with brands,' she said. 'Could we represent you?'

I said yes straight away because I hadn't felt wanted by someone who has access to a work lanyard in a very long time. So I agreed to one organic post every day, plus two ads a week. That was fine when I had something to say, but today I've got nothing and I need Johno home. I need to work out what to post. I need to open every message and make sure everyone feels seen. I need to explain why I wrote about my miscarriage to those who told me it should be kept private. I need to give hope and support to those who have just lost another pregnancy.

I need him to look after our girl, so I can look after these women.

But his work is busy. He is training a new finance assistant. Her name's Eilis Hamilton-Kerr and 'she can barely count,' he told me, but I think he secretly enjoys having a protégé. Or at least one female in his life who does as she's told. I tried to find her on Instagram but could only find an avatar of a sultry brunette pouting to the world. Johno had described her as 'geeky-looking', so I scrolled on.

I look up and Scout is doing a very slow blink. It's 7.00 p.m. and she can barely hold her head up.

'You tired, nugget?'

'No, I'm OK.'

She's lost interest in her ice cream and when she's this tired, it's like she's tiny again. Like those winter days coming back from the park when I would lay her on the sofa and she'd fall asleep in her coat and shoes, mouth open and dreams peaceful. When she's like this, she needs me more.

I carry her upstairs and brush her teeth, but we skip bath-time. I wrap her in clean pyjamas, buttoned up to the top, and her eyes are closing as soon as I pull up the duvet. The toddler years have gone, but some toddler moments remain.

I reach for my phone, but it's downstairs, so I just sit and watch her. I stroke my finger over her nose, like I did when she was tiny. I sweep hair off her forehead and kiss her gently. I whisper in her ear, 'You can do anything,' and she drifts away, with me the last thing she sees.

She is perfect like this, like an infant again.

When Scout was about seven weeks old, I heard a group of girls coming back from a night out. It was 3.00 a.m., I was breastfeeding and one of them stopped to have a piss on the kerb. I could hear the splashes and the laughter and one of them shouting, 'Cazza's got her flaps out again!'

Their laughter bounced off the walls and into our pitch-black room and for a moment I longed to be with them, instead of being alone with this little pink creature that I had longed to be with for so long.

Scout was our miracle, but for a while I was so empty.

My friends were scattered across the country, and I had the baby, so I was left alone. Enjoy your lot. Although, in those early months, my lot made me imagine the sound my body would make hitting a car and I wondered who the driver would be and if I could time it so they missed the buggy. I kept these things to myself, because being a mother is all I've ever wanted.

It filled me completely, but it also took something away.

I watch her a little longer, rest my nose on her hair and take in her scent.

Her nose is shiny, like a little acorn, and I run my index finger gently along the bridge, watching her small, leaden body.

Then I put the landing light on to let a little soft light into her room and very quietly pull out all three drawers from the chest by her bed and tip them onto the floor.

Half of her things are too small and should go, and the rest should be better organised. Leggings and jeans need a space separate to dresses and skirts. Her new uniform needs a drawer of its own. She's too big for these old bodysuits and we might never need them again.

I come across the Babygro we took Scout home in from hospital. It's so small, it looks like it wouldn't cover a hand. I put it to one side and feel tears pushing against my eyelids because our baby was so small.

By the time I hear Johno in the doorway, I'm surrounded by perfectly folded clothes and have started on the box under her bed, with its old breast pump and nappy cream and ointments. He creaks up the stairs.

'Hey,' he says.

'Hi.'

'What are you doing?'

'I'm organising things.'

'Won't you wake Scout?'

'She's fine, she's asleep.'

'I could do this on Saturday?'

'I want to do it now.'

He kneels down to fold a dress that has already been folded.

'It's fine,' I say. 'It's quicker if I do it.'

Then he tries to hug me, but that's not what I need. I need him to be home earlier. I need him to say goodnight to Scout. I smile and don't hug back.

'Are you sure I can't help?'

'It's fine. I'm just tired. Do you think you can leave work on time a bit more next week?'

Silence hangs in the air as he realises the issue, like a cartoon character coming round from a mild concussion. I can almost see the stars hovering over his head.

'It's just things are crazy at the moment. It won't be long, I've just got to get bumped up, show I can do it for six months, then I can slack off like everyone else.'

'I know, but I'm working, too, and we said we'd share it.'

'We will. Definitely.'

He is using what he thinks is his kind voice. It is actually his 'please, wife, don't go mad' voice.

'It's just it's late. It's nearly eight and I haven't posted.'

'It's actually gone nine.'

I need my phone.

I need to post something.

I'm missing the window.

I need to post between 8.00 p.m. and 9.00 p.m., because the algorithm rewards consistency.

Jenn told me this.

I need it to be funny and warm and I haven't had time to think. I need to lift people up and jolt people out of their day-to-day.

And I need to post an ad in two days.

People need uplifting. I need uplifting.

I pick up the old breast pump from a box by my side.

'Johno. Could you take a picture?'

We're at the kitchen table, the pump attached to my right breast, the glare of the ring light in my face. My boobs haven't lactated for three years, but a breast pump is a powerful symbol. I have an open laptop in front of me and have given Johno my phone. He looks confused.

'Like that?'

I smile. 'I'm being empowering.'

When I'm stuck, I remind people: I'm the angry breastfeeding one.

'You'll have to go back a bit,' I say.

He takes a picture and hands my phone back, but the image is no good.

'Maybe try squatting down a little.'

He gets his knees slightly bent and holds the phone horizontally.

'Leave space at the top and bottom for me to crop. Is it square-on?'

'What does that mean?'

'Square – just square. Flat, straight.'

'Yes.'

He takes some, a little more grudgingly, and hands my phone back. They're not quite right. They're a little tilted when they should be perfectly flat.

I take the phone around, and the breast pump bangs the table until I grab it with my other hand. I hold the phone exactly as it needs to be.

'From here.'

He takes the phone, holding it mid-air in exactly the spot I had it.

'It just needs to be perfectly square-on,' I say, and he rolls his eyes like a teenage boy who's been asked to tidy his room.

'I'm not a selfie stick.'

'This is work, too.'

He never accepts this. Never accepts that this is a way to earn a living.

Five minutes of helping puts him in a silent fury. He fixes a blank face as I smile for the pictures because the algorithm promotes smiles.

He hands over the phone and there is one good image and I feel a short wave of relief. I have used my real breastfeeding photos too many times before. I write and upload.

I was made redundant. I walked out of the glass revolving doors and didn't know what to do. I was untethered and unwanted. I sat on a park bench with my box of used notepads, half-chewed biros and the framed photo of baby Scout that I'd stashed away in a drawer. I was discarded for trying to feed my child. But why am I still banging on about this? For all the women who can't say anything for fear of losing their job. For all of us that want to work and earn and have a role alongside being a mother, because that is a job, too. A full-time role. It's not a hobby or a side hustle, it's a privileged position and anyone pushing a mother out of the workforce for pushing out a baby – or trying to feed one – has simply forgotten where they came from #raisingthenextgeneration #maternitydiscrimination
[Disclaimer: I do not still breastfeed or express. I stopped at nine months, though each woman's choice is her own. Fed is best.]

10

DYLAN

Noah is tucked up in bed and on our plates are the leftovers of a Sunday tea of *pommes de terre de toms*: baked spuds with tinned tomatoes. I put Worcestershire sauce in the toms and boil them down so they reduce and get thick and rich, and it costs about 40p a plate. 'ave that, Nigella.

The 'recipe' was my first post for One Day Soon and exactly zero people gave a shit, but it's become our Sunday-night tradition. It's nice and heavy so that he sleeps well.

I wash up and make the place clean, make myself some tea, and as the kettle boils, the scuffed laminate on the kitchen counter glares at me.

I close my eyes and exhale. This weekend was good. We watched films and played in the park and made a little Duplo world. Our time together feels more precious now he's at school.

And my weekdays are better too. I'm getting more calls done, sending *The Women Who Watch On* to more people.

The kettle bubbles and boils. I pour hot water into a mug that says 'H2-Oh that's a nice brew' and sit at the dining table. I roll a fag and lean out the bay window.

73

I allow myself a few rollies a week, once Noah is asleep. It's like prison rations. The first tug makes my head tingle a bit, and I hang out the window to exhale, like a naughty schoolkid. I think this is what the women at the school gates would call mindfulness. That woman who elbowed me is probably frigging off to some Buddhist chant right now.

I look down on the roots of Noah's favourite tree, pushing through the pavement like a giant fist trying to punch through a door. Or like they want to get up and walk away to live in a nice forest. Noah once found an ant crawling up the tree and named it 'Eric' and now every time we walk past, he has to check if Eric is OK.

I shiver a little, pull my cardigan tighter around my shoulders and wonder what to do. It's 9.00 p.m. I could clean, but the flat looks OK. I could watch TV, but everything just shouts too much.

What you watching that shit for, Dilly?

I pick up my phone and flick through Instagram, while my other hand hangs out the window trailing smoke.

I follow a woman called @Mother_minded who has a million followers and posts pictures of herself in flowing dresses and floppy hats alongside inspirational quotes. Her profile says: 'Woman, Mother, Survivor' – though it's not clear what she's survived. But she always wears long sleeves, so maybe she's also got little white ridges like mine; dashes and scars like an emo badge. Like you're all needy and Mummy doesn't care enough and you want to look interesting, when really, sometimes, it's just a way to feel something when your mind's so full it can't feel anything at all.

She's got a new post where she's sitting on a fence in a field, wearing a floaty long-sleeved dress and wellies. She's got this beautiful, natural blonde hair over her shoulders and her figure's so curvy it's like it could move in waves. She looks at the camera and smiles like she knows things about you.

Three years ago I was suffering a severe depressive episode and couldn't care for my own children. Today my book is a number-one bestseller. However bad it gets, give life a chance to get better. Find Your True You at the link in bio.

I scroll through her life. It looks like she lives on a farm now and sells flannels. But mostly what she does is say sad things and hope that people believe them.

I put my phone down.

I should write something.

Give the world something sad about me.

I should write about Dad.

I get my laptop from the counter, sit on the sofa and log in to One Day Soon. The views counter hasn't moved.

I stare at the screen and very slowly type.

One Day Soon
22:17, 16 September

The Man on the Southbound Platform
When Mum told me about Dad, I was watching *Animal Planet*.

It was an autumn evening and dark outside and she came into the room and turned the telly off.

'I'm watching that!'

I was thirteen and enraged by everything.

But she looked as if flicking that switch was the hardest decision she'd ever made.

Then she opened her mouth and something stuck, and this noise came out of her. Like a little moan stopped halfway and she had to pull it back in and said, 'Your dad's dead.'

Like she was saying, 'Dinner's ready.'

Not, 'There's something I've got to tell you.'

Not even, 'I've got bad news.'

Just, 'Your dad's dead.'

He's dust, move on.

And then she cried so much I knew it was true, and she wrapped herself around me and her body shook and I just stared at the black telly screen and looked at us both in the reflection.

She said he died on the platform at Balham, but that wasn't true. And I think she told me that because she was ashamed.

Ashamed that she was the grown-up, and she didn't do enough to help him.

Because really, he died on the tracks.

He finished work, had a drink and got the 20:11 to Sutton, but sometimes you have to change.

So he got off, and the platform was busy, and he walked to the far end and stepped in front of a fast one to Gatwick.

She didn't tell me that, but you get to hear it anyway. There are news reports. It becomes whispered in the playground, and girls will make sure that you know too.

And I'll wonder what he was thinking just before.

Like, was he thinking about me and Mum, or was he so sad there was nothing in his head at all?

Or maybe he just looked up at the pigeon spikes and thought, 'Well, that's enough.'

I want him to tell me why it had to be then.

I want to know why he made it halfway home.

*

76

It's Monday afternoon and the kids all come out clutching paintings, their bags dwarfing their little bodies. Noah's class isn't first and that's OK, but it isn't second either and I need to get home for some follow-up calls.

When Ms Carole comes out, I step forward a bit, but he's still not there.

Why hasn't she noticed?

How long has he been gone?

And then I see him right at the back and my shoulders drop and my muscles ease. I wave my hand, but he doesn't see me.

His little jacket is hanging down his back and off his shoulders, and he's pretending to be a penguin. He's pretending to waddle about, his feet and hands turned out to the side, while a little girl next to him does an exaggerated laugh. She's a tiny bit taller than him, with big brown eyes and perfect blonde plaits. Then she joins in with the waddling, and he cackles like an old barmaid.

'Noh! Noah!'

But he's in his own world with this girl and I'm being blanked by my own son.

'Noah!'

I shout, a bit too loud, and get side-eye from the mum next to me. Finally Noah sees me and waves back. He reaches up to the sky with one arm, so Ms Carole knows he's ready to go, and stares at her like a well-trained Collie. She nods, he runs to me and I bend down to wrap around him and for a moment it's just us.

And then he pushes me away.

'Mummy, did you see me be a penguin?'

'Yes, I did.'

'It's like this.'

He gives me a demo of penguin-ing.

'That's great, Noh.'

'Mummy, can I play with Scout today?'

'Who's Scout?'

'She's my friend!'

He says this like I'm an idiot. Like knowing who Scout is should be as simple as understanding that rain is wet.

He drags me a few steps towards the girl from the back of the queue, who is talking to a man who I guess is her dad. He's holding a PAW Patrol lunch box like it's a diamanté clutch bag and wearing smart jeans and white trainers. He might have looked good once but now has the energy of an old tangerine in the bottom of a school bag.

The little girl, Scout, is giving him the big eyes, speaking in a soft voice.

'Daddy, can Noah come and play at our house?'

Then Noah joins in.

'Can I, Mummy? Letitia and Mary have playdates all the time.'

I don't know who Letitia and Mary are, and I don't know when he learned the word 'playdate', but I know I'm not going to this man's house. I need to get back for the last hour of calling.

'Not today, Noh, I've got to work.'

'But, Mummy, please?'

'Please can he, Daddy?'

'Umm, well, I don't know, Scouty. It sounds like his mummy's working, so maybe another time.'

The dad looks at me like there is some shared understanding between us. He smiles gently. Our kids look forlorn for a second, and Noah tries again.

'But, Mummy, I really want to.'

'Noah, not today.'

'Oh, Mummy, please! That's so unfair! I'm *never* allowed to play!'

His face goes bright red and his eyes water. It's a scream out of nowhere. But we play all the time. I love playing with him.

'*Please*, Mummy.'

He crosses his arms and looks up at me.

'I said, no.'

I don't want to go to this man's home. I can't remember the last time I had to speak to a man outside of work calls.

'But I want to!'

'No!'

I say it too loudly. Noah flinches and I regret it, because now this playground dad thinks I shout at my child.

'Maybe another day, Scout,' the man says, trying to deflate things. He says it like he's helping and turns to face me. 'I'm Johno.'

He stretches out a hand, which seems very formal as we're surrounded by kids demanding Dairylea Dunkers, but we shake and now I have to tell him who I am, because that's the deal, isn't it? Smile, greet, serve information to strangers.

'Dylan. Noah's mum.'

'I guessed, as they sent him your way. Although, given the chaos, I wouldn't blame them if they lost one or two a year.'

He grins at this, because children being kidnapped is hilarious, of course.

'It's no bother if Noah does want to come back. I can give him tea at ours if you want? If you're nearby I could bring him back to you for six-ish?'

What is he on? I've met him twelve seconds ago and now he wants to make off with my son?

'It's OK. He'll be tired.'

'I'm not, Mummy.'

'Noah . . .'

I use my stern voice. I feel my lungs tighten and I just want to leave now.

'Thank you,' I say to Johno, 'but we should go.'

'No problem. Come on, Scouty, let's leave Dylan and Noah alone now.'

He begins to walk off and I do, too. But then I realise we'll be strolling across the playground together in silence, so I just stop. Noah looks confused. Maybe I didn't need to be so off with Johno.

'Nice to meet you,' I say, and give him a smile.

'And you.'

He smiles back and walks on, and his daughter waves at Noah, before reaching for her father's hand.

Maybe I'm being ridiculous. This man is normal, isn't he? Nice. He's carrying a PAW Patrol lunch box and his eyes look safe. But then, Ted Bundy had kind eyes and he bludgeoned women as they slept.

I crouch down to speak to my boy.

'Sorry, Noah, but I've got to finish off some calls. Maybe another day, OK?'

His eyes are watering and he can barely look at me.

'But you didn't have to come. You'll just be working and it's boring.'

'You can't go to strangers' houses on your own, darling.'

'But it's not a stranger, she's my friend.'

He's lost. Distraught. He thinks I'm being cruel to him for the fun of it and it makes my heart break.

'But look, Noh, her dad's a stranger, isn't he? And we have to be careful with strangers.'

'But you never let me have any friends!'

He shouts this time, and a few lingering mums turn their heads. One smiles at me.

'Noah, that's not true. I just have to work. You'll have a play-date another time.'

'Promise?'

'I promise.'

He mulls this over like he's a master negotiator.

I make my last stab at a deal. 'How about you have tea in front of the telly tonight?'

He nods, like this will be a real help. The very least I can do.

We begin to walk home, but his hand is limp in mine. As we get out of the gate, this pent-up breath comes out of me like I'm deflating and I don't know what's wrong with me.

The girl was nice and her dad had a kind face and cared about his daughter's friendships and I just need to breathe a bit more. This was always going to happen. It's good that it happens.

My son has made a friend. She makes him laugh.

And her dad will not put his hand to my neck and scream in my face.

I inhale and exhale, let it all flow out.

He was just being nice. He was kind to his girl, friendly to me, and maybe he just wanted to help. Maybe he's on his own, too, so he understands. I didn't see his wedding finger, but he didn't mention a wife.

And he tried to make me laugh. His little joke about losing kids. It wasn't funny, but he tried to make me laugh and no one else does that.

As we walk home, Noah's hand stays limp and he still speaks in his sad voice.

'Mummy?'

'Yes?'

'Will I ever be allowed to have playdates?'

'Of course. We'll just have to plan it next time.'

'But I can have one? With my friend Scout?'

'Definitely.'

'Tomorrow?'

'Very soon, I promise. I'll talk to her daddy.'

I give him a peck on the forehead and stroke his hair.

My little boy needs friends.

11
LO

It's the Thursday school run, I'm nose to my phone in a corner of the playground and I can't believe it's taken three weeks to take a look at this.

The home page of the Influenza forum is magenta and grey and looks like an interface from an 80s Commodore. There are no images, no fancy fonts, no design. Just reams of anonymous users with fake avatars and the 'viewing' numbers are staggering. There are currently 13,567 people viewing a thread about @Mother_minded: a mental-health advocate with one million followers, who promotes wellness retreats and lavender flannels. Someone announces she is universally hated at her kids' school. There's a screen grab of @Mother_minded's wrist and someone has noticed a faint scar.

Mileycyprus says: I wish she would finish the job and do us all a favour.

Kalabash says: Jeez, are you serious? We can joke, but that crosses the line.

Mileycyprus says: Is that you @Mother_minded? Lol.

Jade1974 says: Kalabash is right, that's too much. But if you put yourself out there, you've got to accept people will talk.

Sisterpledge says: It's her kids I feel most sorry for. Imagine being eighteen and your mates finding pictures of your shitting arse have been splashed all over the internet?

Motherofhaggins says: Love you guys. You make me feel sane. I have severe PND and every time I see people like her pretending to be my friend while telling me I need a £20 lavender-scented flannel I feel like I'm failing.

The responses come within minutes, sometimes seconds. It's a living, breathing corner of the internet. Influenza's bio reads: 'Gossip has been around for centuries'.

But gossip was over a garden fence or down the pub, not shared with 13,567 people.

There are hundreds of threads, on everything from influencers to Moon-landing conspiracies. It's a river of consciousness, gathering sticks and unsettling stones along the way, and I can't stop reading.

Then I see it: 'The Lo Down'. My heart tightens. I click through. Even though it's about me, it feels invasive, like I'm peering through a gap in the fence into someone else's garden. There are three month-old comments.

Mushypeasplease says: Thoughts? At least she has a cause, unlike the rest of them?

Tedsmum says: Yeah, don't mind her. She also doesn't block anyone who disagrees with her. She just needs to stop parading her kid about on the internet.

Chumley_corner says: Like her.

I feel like I've been promoted. Like someone has verified me. They like me.

84

An advert for nappies suddenly cuts through the magenta screen, a tiny, smiling infant in a perfect grey living room, and my mind flits to the emptiness of my womb.

A cacophony of kids jolts me out of Influenza and I look up. I'm standing next to a giant metal bin as other parents gather nearby. There is the first hint of orange coming across the leaves on the big oak tree next to the playground and Ms Carole has her arm around a little girl with immaculate braids.

I put my phone in my pocket and feel the heat on my thigh. This is my favourite part of the day. It's a kind of night-before-Christmas excitement that builds over six hours until our eyes lock together and Scout runs to me, her hand slips into mine and we walk away, two halves of the same walnut.

I spot her. She is chatting conspiratorially to a boy with a brown bowl cut and hasn't seen me. Wisps of hair are jutting out at odd angles from her pigtails and there's a bronze sticker on her jumper.

I start waving at her, grinning manically. I'm not sure if I look endearing or terrifying, but I want Scout's attention. When she spots me, she grins back and begins jumping up and down, stretching her arm up to the sky. For some reason, I start jumping too, forgetting that I'm with other adults. I feel a woman to my right edge slightly past me to get a clear view of her kid. I wonder if the parents should have a line, too.

'Mummy!'

She's released by Ms Carole and thunders towards me.

'Nugget!'

I kneel down and hug her until I can feel her tiny ribcage. Everyone dissolves around us and I inhale the end-of-day scent of her.

'Can I have a snack?'

I pull a clear pouch of crustless Marmite sandwiches from my bag. She pulls a face but takes them when I offer a banana as an alternative, which she looks at like a recently severed pig's ear.

Hand in hand, we walk over a rainbow painted on the playground tarmac and out of the red iron gates, weaving in and out of buggies. We walk around two chatting dads clogging up the pavement until we are at the zebra crossing. The lollipop lady sternly gestures for a Deliveroo driver to let the next generation pass.

'Can we go to the park?'

Scout mumbles half the sentence as she remembers, midchew, not to speak with her mouth full.

'I've got to get back and do a bit of work, Scout.'

For every ad partnership that lands, there are twenty pitches that don't and they take time and thought. I also have subtitles to add to the latest Etisk video, because the client is chasing and needs it ASAP. Those ethically sourced Scandinavian dungarees won't sell themselves.

But this is becoming a familiar argument with Scout, like the one this morning about not wearing neon pink socks to school.

'Everyone else is going to the park,' she counters.

She knows my weak spot is other parents doing more than me. I think she's known since she arrived in the world that I'd do anything to make her happy. Babies learn it, just like puppies – same head tilt, eyes made large. And now she can speak, she has refined it and knows just how to play the right heartstrings.

'Another day, Scout.'

I hold her hand as we cross the road. She says nothing as we amble, me holding her book bag and lunch box, her begrudgingly holding my hand like it's an unwanted toy.

'So, how was your day?' I ask, determined to distract.

'Good.'

'What was good about it?'

'It was just good.'

'Who did you play with?'

'Noah,' she says. 'He's in the park now.'

We continue in silence, both turning our heads towards a sapling tree with what looks like a whole box of cornflakes scattered at its roots. Normally, Scout would have questions about why the cornflakes were on the floor or who put them there, but she remains quiet as we sidestep the orange explosion, her hand slipping out of mine.

I stop in the middle of the pavement. I can add subtitles this evening. It's just work, and this is Scout. I do this job to be with her, not to make her watch me tap on a laptop.

She looks at me. I smile.

'Come on, then.'

'Really?'

She's back to herself in an instant, hope bursting across her face. I nod and grin.

'Thank you, Mummy!'

She squeals and squeezes my hand.

She has a friend and he might be someone she has sleepovers with, someone she tells secrets to. This could be a pal she eats cake with in a den made of clothes horses and old sheets. This might be a memory.

I have time.

The park has two metal barriers at the entrance, to stop people driving through. Scout swings underneath one and propels herself towards the inner playground gates.

'There he is,' she squeals, pointing to the little boy from the line at school. Joy spills out of her face and I feel a surge of happiness wash over me and a twinge of sadness that her frothiness is not for me. I wonder what the moment was when they felt the warmth of friendship seep over them. Was it over a shared paint pot? Singing, 'The ink is black, the page is white' in assembly?

She jiggles impatiently from foot to foot as I try to open the iron gate with my pinkie finger, the rest of my digits burdened with her lunch box and water bottle and my bag.

It swings open; I turn around to close it, turn back to Scout to ask if she wants a drink and she's gone. She's run over to the boy and they're careening around like foals released into the wild.

I imagined having school-mum friends. Perhaps a circle of women who would help with pick-ups and collectively groan about homework. But I hadn't factored in how to make them.

On the graffitied bench are two women in denim dungarees showing each other their phones as their toddlers sit in a nearby sandpit. Two dads stand apart under an oak tree with their arms crossed as their sons pound up the metal slide.

There's the angry woman from the school playground, leaning against the slide. She has cropped, peroxide hair and jet-black roots, and is frowning into her phone. Over her denim jeggings, she wears an oversized black cardigan, and on her delicate feet, battered white plimsolls.

I put Scout's things down next to a patch of weeds. Scout is on a tractor-shaped metal frame on a giant spring, which Noah pushes quite violently. They're making a sound that's part pterodactyl, part monkey. I look around to see which one is his parent. I should introduce myself to the little boy who is making my daughter squeal with laughter.

'Hi, are you Noah?'

I take the tone of a primary-school teacher and wonder what the etiquette is of introducing yourself to a stranger's child.

'Yes.'

He immediately stops pushing the tractor frame. He has big blue eyes and thick brown hair cut to a neat fringe. You can almost picture him sitting there as his mum snips across with the kitchen scissors.

Then the peroxide-blonde woman in the jeggings starts marching over. She looks like a sunken-eyed model of the 90s. There's an intensity to her that makes me step back.

Scout's eyes plead for me to go away, which breaks my heart and fills it at the same moment.

'Mummy, can we play now?'

'OK, Scout.'

The mum arrives and speaks to the boy, ignoring me.

'Are you OK, Noh?'

Of course he's OK. What does she think I'm doing? I give her my best smile.

'Are you Noah's mum?'

'Yes.'

She sounds like she's staking a claim. Or making an accusation. So much defensiveness in one little word. She tucks her phone into her pocket and crosses her arms over her torso. Based on my face or my clothes or my daughter, she's decided something about me. I don't know what it is, but she doesn't like it.

She's wearing a tight, white long-sleeved tee under her cardigan and it shows the shape of her breasts. She would pass the pencil test. We're about the same height, but somehow she looks small. Like a fierce pixie.

'Hi, I'm Lo.' I wave, even though we're only a few feet apart, and she nods back.

'Hi.'

She doesn't give me her name. Her nails are red raw and peeling from being bitten too close. She sees me looking and recrosses her arms and looks down at the kids as they play. She stares at them both like she's doing a crossword and shouldn't be interrupted. Like I've already disrupted things enough.

I look her way, to see if she'll make eye contact. My mum told me I had a habit of staring at people until the whole room was uncomfortable, so I get my phone out to check if Johno has messaged. He hasn't. I skim across to Influenza – 123 new comments on the @Mother_minded thread, but nothing new on me. I put the phone back. Scout is now jiggling the tractor as Noah throws his arms around as though he might fall off.

'Ride 'em cowboy,' I say, which everyone ignores.

I've never been able to sit or stand in silence. Silence is not golden, it's an uncomfortable void that I always fill. I once told the owner of our local corner shop that I had a bladder infection while buying a bag of frozen cranberries. She'd just asked for two quid.

'I'm Scout's mum,' I say.

She nods like I've told her the capital of France is Paris and gives the briefest upturn to her lips. She's standing at a distance, huddled in her cardigan like its armour.

'Yes,' she says, 'I've met your husband.'

'Oh. When? I don't think I've seen you before at school. Do you pick Noah up?'

'Yes, I pick him up.'

Maybe she's shy. But there's shy and there's rude. If you've met my husband, then you know who I am.

I turn my gaze towards the kids, who are now jumping into a small puddle and jousting with soggy, chestnut-tree leaves.

I've always got on better with boys. Amara once drunkenly said, 'I really didn't like you *at all* when I met you.' She stressed the 'at all' like it was a compliment. 'You were just so bloody *cheery*, and confident, and fucking . . . *friendly* all the time.'

Then she gave me a hug and a wet kiss on the forehead.

So, I stand there, holding my phone like it's a stress ball, and hope this mum says something before I do.

The silence lingers. Then she looks at me.

'I passed you in Asda, you were rushing somewhere,' she says, before turning to the kids and shouting, 'Noah, share, please. Give the stick to Scout.'

It feels strange hearing a stranger shout Scout's name. I don't know her, but she knows my daughter and my husband. I try to remember her, but I can't. I'd remember icy blonde hair and jet-black roots. All I can remember is the soap dispenser and the blood.

'How funny, I don't remember, but maybe it was me,' I say, realising it's not funny at all.

'You were wearing that yellow mac. It's easy to remember. Right, Noah, we need to get going, come on.'

Her son looks appalled.

'What?'

The kids have only just begun to play. Why is she so desperate to get away?

'Sorry, I didn't ask your name,' I say. 'I don't know about you, but I'm relieved to no longer be called "Scout's mum" at nursery. It's good to be Lo again.'

She smiles an empty smile.

'Dyl,' she says, taking a few steps away to gather Noah's bag, 'short for Dylan.' I want to say something about Bob Dylan or Dylan from *The Magic Roundabout*, but decide against it.

Dyl wraps Noah in a blue duffel coat as I call Scout to me. She flashes another half-smile at us and starts heading towards the gate, towing him behind her.

'But I don't want to go!'

He looks distraught.

'Nice to meet you,' Dyl says over her shoulder, but I'm not sure she means it.

I look at Scout's face: she has deflated again, her play ended as soon as it began. They've only been there for two minutes.

Dyl must want to get away from me, which makes me feel empty too. I don't think I was too chatty; I don't think I told her enough about me to want to walk away. And, anyway, Scout has a human she's found outside of our family. Noah could be someone who laughs at her jokes and stands up for her in the playground. This isn't about us.

'Does Noah want to come to tea?'

I blurt it out like I'm calling for Scout to stop at the kerb. The kids gasp. Dyl looks at me like I've asked for a threesome. She goes to say something, but Noah interrupts.

'Please, Mummy, you promised we could! Remember?'

I don't know what he means, but I realise I've probably made her dislike me even more. It's too late, and she knows it, and so I have nothing to lose.

'It's no problem, we're just round the corner,' I continue, slightly more bullish. I want to prove this woman wrong. She's misjudged me. I'll get her to like me because Scout likes Noah. 'And they've hardly had any time to play.'

Noah lowers his voice and says, 'Pleeeeease.'

Scout claps her hands together and puts a big closed-lip smile across her face. She stands perfectly upright, like the soldier on a cuckoo clock.

'Please, Mummy,' says Noah. 'I really want to. Just once! Really quickly!' He too is making his eyes large. 'I've never been to anyone's house before.'

These tiny manipulators know where to get us all.

'You have, Noh,' she says, her tone a bit defensive.

'Not to play.'

And it's about the saddest thing I've ever heard. What four-year-old has never had a playdate?

'OK,' she says, looking down at her boy. 'But we can't stay long.'

The kids shout, 'Yay!'

'Ohmigosh we can play dress up,' says Scout.

And finally, this mother has to really look me in the eye.

'I have to work later, so we can't stay long. Shall I get anything along the way?'

'No, no: I've got all we need.'

I smile and we walk off in silence.

12

DYLAN

Lo opens the door and the hallway smells of lavender. Like a Victorian terrace is supposed to feel like the Dordogne or something. Her house looks almost exactly the same as ours from the front: the same bay windows, same old brickwork, but they have it all to themselves and ours is chopped in half, with Mrs Younis below.

London likes to remind you what you don't have. Six months after Dad died, me and Mum moved from a house with a bright blue door to a little flat with dirty white walls, and across the street I could see houses just like the one we'd left behind. Same open porch, same bay windows, just not for us anymore.

'Shoes there, kids,' says Lo.

Scout takes hers off and puts them on a little stand in the hall and Noah copies her and I wonder if I have to as well. I've got a hole in my pop sock and can feel my middle toe pushing through.

But Lo steps into the lounge without removing hers. The floor is all bare wooden boards, buffed and varnished, so there's no carpet to stain. Up the stairwell are pictures of them, hung tightly together to remind anyone who enters how happy they are with their life choices.

There are no doors on the frames, so it all feels open, and the walls are in the same dark 'Hague Blue' that all the other mums on social like. The same women who have 'adult headaches' instead of hangovers, and call vaginas 'fannies' to be cool.

Of all the kids you had to pick, Noh, why did it have to be hers? The woman with the giant yellow mac and the nice husband and the sharp elbows.

I stand, waiting for instruction. The place is immaculate, like she's expecting an estate agent to come round to take photos. It's like something off one of the interiors accounts. There are shutters half open inside the front window, an old Victorian fireplace with deep green tiles, a stack of clean logs and no grate to burn them in. There's a pile of parcels by an old desk, her own private sorting office, and I wonder what she sells.

Noah and Scout are already thundering about upstairs and we stand in silence; two strangers whose kids are singing, 'Let it Go' to the beat of a lightsaber.

'Well, they're having fun,' says Lo.

'Yes.'

We stand and face each other, because our kids are friends and so I have to be in her home.

'What a lovely place you've got.'

'Thanks. It took a bit of fixing. There was a real old-dead-lady vibe when we first moved in. All swirly pub carpets and everything painted peach!'

She smiles as she says this. I have nothing to add, no renovation chat of my own. I don't decorate, because I never know how long we're staying. I smile at her again.

'It's a really beautiful blue.'

'Thanks.'

On the mantelpiece is a vase of fake peonies, one with a missing head, and I wonder if I can start a conversation about that. Anything that means we're not just staring at each other and smiling. But she beats me to it.

'Do you like beauty products?'

I'm not sure why she's asking. Maybe she thinks I need some?

'Yeah, sometimes. I mean, I try not to, because of the environment.'

She looks pale, like she's done something terrible.

'Oh, yes, of course. These are all cruelty-free.'

She puts her phone on the desk, bends down and starts riffling through the open parcels by her desk, each addressed to her in thick, black marker pen or gold italic scrawl.

'And zero waste, some of it. They keep sending it for work, but I can't use most of it. Do you want anything? It's going to the beauty bank otherwise.'

Am I supposed to take these things, these cast-offs? She's nearly knocked me over twice and didn't care, and now she wants to dish out make-up like we're old mates. It's weird.

'What's a beauty bank?'

'They collect unused beauty products for poorer women. Like if you're on the dole and have a job interview.'

She softens the word 'poorer' and looks down, like she shouldn't have said it. Has she decided that already? Is it my roots? My clothes? The lines under my eyes? *Do have this blusher to stop troubling people with your poor face.*

'Aw, thanks, but I don't think I need anything. Let's keep it for the poor women.' I feel charged, suddenly. The muscles around my heart get tight. 'And it's called Jobseeker's Allowance now, not the dole,' I add.

'Yes! Dole's so old-school!'

She smiles but she's embarrassed, says 'old-school' like she's describing retro furniture. And then she turns to go through her stash of products so I can't read her face. The stuff must be worth hundreds.

I can hear Scout telling Noah upstairs that he's 'now Olaf'. As Lo riffles through the parcels, I look at the cluster of framed family photos on her desk. Her and Johno and Scout by the Thames, on a country walk; a foreign beach; next to a wonky snowman; more joy on display and she sifts her pile of swag.

'I'll have to drop this off this week,' she says. 'It's been building up for ages and it's just going to waste.'

'Do you work in beauty, then?'

'Social media,' she says.

'Oh. I thought you must do beauty therapy or something.'

'No.'

She's ripping open a metallic-pink package as confetti flutters to the floor. She holds up a leopard-print make-up bag that says 'You got this babe' and scatters fifteen lipsticks of differing shades onto the desk.

'Wow. Not sure canary yellow will help anyone.' She smirks.

'What do you do in social media?'

'I write about motherhood.'

I wonder what makes one woman more of an authority than another and why that would need fifteen shades of lipstick.

I write about motherhood. It doesn't need lipstick.

'More specifically, the motherhood penalty,' she says, her voice getting harder. 'And women getting fucked over for, well, getting fucked and having a baby.'

The swearing is a tiny performance. Like she's decided she needs to say the bad words to get me on side. Prove that she is not someone who applies lipstick for money.

'They're literally mother fuckers.' She laughs and I smile

back, because the alternative is to stare quietly at fake flowers. I'm not really sure who she's talking about.

'Who are, sorry?'

'The system. Employers.'

Oh. The *system*. Bloody *system* ruins everything.

'You know,' she continues, 'it's like you spend your life working hard on your ABCs, working hard in your GCSEs, working hard in your A-levels . . .'

I want to tell her I didn't get that far, but she's building to a crescendo like she's Martin Luther King.

'. . . Then it's get a job, marry the man, have a baby. Then you lose everything, including yourself, because employers don't want mothers in the workplace.'

She leaves a silence, like she's waiting for applause. It feels like she normally gets it. Like she's running off a script.

'Yes. It's hard for everyone.'

'Yes, of course.'

She stops, like a question is sitting just inside her lips but she's not sure if she's allowed to ask.

There's a thud from upstairs as one of our kids lands on the floorboards. We both pause to listen, waiting for tears or laughter, and then they scream happily and there's a rumble of feet running along the landing.

'Sounds like they're having fun,' Lo says, again.

'Yes,' I smile. 'So who do you write for, when you write about motherhood?'

'It's Instagram, mostly.'

'You work at Instagram?'

'No, on Instagram. I have an account called The Lo Down. That's where I write about motherhood.'

'Oh. Like, full-time?'

'Well, I do some panels, events.'

'So you're an influencer?'

'Kind of. An influencer is just someone who champions something they believe in, but it feels like a dirty word.'

I smile at her, because it all makes sense now. She has an Instagram account and people send her free things. I have a blog and spambots send me porn links. I pull out my phone.

'I follow some of them. Like @Mother_minded.'

'Yes, she's lovely.' She nods a bit but leaves it there.

'Can I have a look?'

'Sure.'

She smiles politely, like it's silly, but I think she's proud. I find her account and maybe she should be. She has 49,500 followers and her life is beautiful. Even more beautiful than in reality, standing in her house.

'Oh, wow, is this you?'

I show her my phone to check, but of course it is. There are pictures of her across the feed. But still I check, as though there might be another person with her face, and daughter, and green velvet sofa.

'Yeah,' she says, 'but it's not really me, I suppose. No one can be human in a photo and a 300-word caption.'

'And this is how you work?'

'Yes.'

'How does it earn money, though?'

She's a bit shocked, like I'm not supposed to ask.

'Well, you build an audience and then brands ask you to do ads.'

Just like that. Build an audience and free things follow.

'I mean, I mostly flog bog roll,' she says, rolling her eyes a bit.

She's being self-deprecating, talking herself down to make me feel better as I scroll through her life. There she is swinging Scout upside down, there she is looking sternly at the camera.

There she is in this very room, with a jumper stuck halfway over her head while Scout does the same thing. And there's her with Johno, a flashback to her wedding day, looking like she's won the great cock raffle of 2012.

I drift into her world for a moment, every pixel, every perfect square, every cause and bit of family goofing, while the real thing stands limply next to me.

'It can be a very powerful platform,' she says.

The kids stampede downstairs and through the lounge, the rush lifting a few pieces of confetti from the desk where Lo had neatly scooped them up. Noah runs around me and into the kitchen. We're just obstacles in their game now.

'Noh, come here quickly.'

He pretends not to hear me.

'C'mon, Noh, over here now,' I say, a little firmer. 'Let me look at your face. What's that on your cheek?'

'It's a PAW Patrol stamp,' he says, as I go to rub it off. 'No, please can I keep it on? It's our stamp to get back into the cinema.'

I pause just long enough for him to run off to watch a film with Scout that only exists in their minds.

Lo folds the empty packaging under her arm and gestures with her elbow towards the kitchen.

'That's it, they don't need us anymore,' she smiles. 'Fancy a brew?'

She walks through to the open-plan kitchen, drops the flattened boxes by the bin and pulls a packet of kettle chips from a floor-to-ceiling food cupboard.

Or maybe when they're that big they get called larders.

The kitchen is new, but is styled to look old. Like it came from Victorian times but with built-in white goods. She empties the crisps into a bowl, turns the kettle on, then pulls back a chair to sit at the wooden six-person kitchen table, and I do the same.

'So, what do you do? For work, I mean. Obviously, mumming is full-time,' she says.

'I'm a writer, too.'

I say it, then feel like an idiot, because I don't know if I'm ready to talk about my work with someone who thinks you can change a woman's life with Sunset Blush lipstick.

'But I pay the bills with telesales,' I add.

'What do you write about?'

'Myself.'

'Well,' she says, 'write what you know, eh?'

She smiles and I realise, as I sit in this stranger's home, that if our kids stay friends, I'm probably going to have to let her into mine too. She will see the landlord-supplied sofa that has been worn down by many arses. She will know there are stubborn black spots of damp in the corner of the living-room window, where the water sits on the wood inside the single pane. She will see that the countertop is laminated chipboard and has yellow duct tape over the bit where it meets the sink to stop water rotting away the area where the lamination has cracked off. I change this tape regularly, but she won't know that and if I tell her, she'll think I'm mad because why would you tell anyone that?

'And where do you write?'

'On the sofa, mostly.'

She laughs, but I wasn't joking.

'No, I mean, who for? Where does it go?'

'Just for me.'

That's not true, of course. But I don't want to wave my non-moving views counter at a woman with 49,500 followers.

'Oh, cool. Would you ever want to send your stuff to anyone?'

'No.'

And, of course, that's not true either, but it stops her for a moment and I change the subject.

'Lo is such a pretty name. I don't think I've heard it before.'

'It's short for Lois, which is pretty short already.'

I smile at her and we both sit and take turns deliberately reaching for crisps and for a moment the room is silent but for the crunching of fried spuds dusted in rosemary.

'These are nice.'

'Yes,' she says, 'I'm addicted.'

On the wall is a corkboard full of loose photos and invites: memories made and memories yet to happen. There's a picture of Johno there too. It's recent, but he looks fresher than in the playground. He's somewhere warm, in a pale shirt with this big smile. A full, open, happy-with-all-things smile. He looks like a man who would make sure that things work, and I wonder what it must be like to raise a kid with someone like that.

Below it is one with Scout and an older boy of about eight.

'Does Scout have a brother?'

'No, that's a friend's kid. We haven't seen them for ages. We just have the one.'

I want to ask if they'll have another, because I'd like to talk about anything that isn't me or crisps, but I also don't want to quiz her on what she's doing with her genitals. But she tells me anyway.

'We want another one,' she says. 'It hasn't happened yet.'

'It can take a while.'

'It's recurrent miscarriage for us. I have a heart-shaped uterus, which means the egg can't always attach to the uterus wall.'

She tells me like I'll have heard of it and know an easy way to fix it and I don't quite know what to say to her.

'Sorry,' she says. 'I probably shouldn't have shared that with a stranger. Me and my heart-shaped uterus!'

And then she makes a heart shape with her hands, and stands to rip some kitchen towel off a roll and sweep up crisp crumbs from the table.

I've never known anyone just say things like that.

How close must it be to the surface if it bubbles up to someone you've just met? Why doesn't she talk about it to friends? It's like she needs a dab of warmth from somewhere.

'I'm really sorry,' I say.

'No, look it's fine. Insta can make you a bit too open sometimes. I'm so used to telling everyone everything. Hey guys, have a look at my heart-shaped uterus!'

She smiles, and maybe I need an empathy injection and to stop being such a snarky cow.

'Well, I hope you are OK.'

'Yes of course. People deal with much worse. And, hey, there are days when one kid is definitely enough.'

She says this with a big wide grin, but it feels like performance again and she shifts things on.

'Where did you have Noah?'

'Haringey General.'

'No way! Scout was born on Broxton ward.'

'Noah, too!'

I'm not sure why my voice is suddenly so high, but we're just glad to be talking about something else.

'So, are you from here then?'

'No,' I tell her, 'but I've moved around the area a bit.'

'Wait,' she says. 'When was he born?'

'Twelfth of May.'

'Oh, wow! Scout was the nineteenth!'

'We must've just missed each other.'

'Like ships in the night. Or sows in the yard. You wouldn't have wanted to see me then, to be honest. I had a C-section and it does some weird stuff to your insides: I farted so loudly that night, the woman in the next bed asked to be moved.'

I smile.

'Noah was Caesarean, too. It's pretty undignified. I remember being lowered onto the toilet afterwards by a nurse and shouting, "Am I over the pan, am I over the pan?"'

'Ha!' She lets out this giant laugh. So loud I jolt a bit. I have never told anyone that, and don't know why I told her. But her face is excited, like a puppy with a ball, and she's suddenly got a sparkle in her eyes and for a moment it feels nice to know I can do that to someone. Her openness is contagious.

'Broxton, though,' I say. 'That place is etched in my head forever. I wake up and I can still see the signs pointing down the hospital corridor: BROXTON!'

'There was a couple on the other side of us as we waited to go into theatre,' she says. 'And all you could hear was her contracting and him wriggling in his chair, going, "Well, I guess NHS funds don't go on seating," and she just screamed, "Get the fuck out, Nigel," and threw a bedpan at him.'

'A dry one?'

'Luckily, yes.'

'That's the one advantage to giving birth alone,' I say, and wish I hadn't, because it prompts questions.

But this woman is maybe warmer than I thought, and when she tells you things, you want to tell her things back, and all day long I speak to Noah about cartoons and to faceless office managers about water coolers and vending machines.

'That must've been hard. Johno was useless, but at least he was there.'

She wants to ask more, I think, but then the kids come running in to interrupt us.

'Mummy,' says Scout, 'did you get the drawing paper?'

Scout leans forward to take a crisp without asking.

'Sorry, Scout, I completely forgot.'

Lo's voice is full-on drama club. She looks her daughter straight in the eyes when she speaks and then wraps an arm around her, pulling her under her wing.

'Mummy! I wanted to do it now with Noah.'

'Well, it's OK, it's playtime now, not school time. You and me can do it next week.'

'But you're allowed to do teams.'

'OK, well, I'll try to get some paper soon.'

Lo looks at me and rolls her eyes.

'Oh my God, this project. I swear it's more homework for us than it is the kids.'

I smile gently.

'What project?'

'The autumn project. About harvest.'

'Noah, what's that?'

He's staring at the crisps with a face like he's been caught shoplifting.

'We've got to do a making project at home about harvest, but it can be whatever you want, like pasta and glue or curly paper.'

'Why didn't you tell me?'

He shrugs blankly and looks exactly like his father. It's a look that says: *this is your fault.*

'I forgot?'

'Honestly,' says Lo, 'if I didn't search Scout's bag every night I'd never know anything. You're not great at passing on notes, are you, Scout? We didn't even know about the school photos.'

Her daughter shrugs, too, but with a sideways smile for her mum.

'What photos?' I ask.

'They had a photographer in. We missed that note, which is why she looks such a scruff.'

She nods to the corkboard and there is Scout, perfectly presented in her school cardigan, plaits immaculate, smile fixed for the camera.

'When did that happen?'

'First week, I think.'

'But I didn't give permission.'

'Oh. Well, I think they just delete them if you don't want them, so it's probably fine.'

'Noah, did you have a photo taken?'

'Yeah,' he says. 'Everyone did.'

'Mummy,' Scout interrupts. 'We can do the project together!'

Noah nearly squeals.

'Yeah!'

'You're allowed to do teams!'

Lo looks at me.

'I mean, it kind of halves the workload,' she says.

'What do they have to do?'

'Draw some cows, maybe? Slap a bit of dried macaroni on some cardboard?'

I don't know anything. I don't know anything about my boy and his life and his schoolwork and who's taking pictures of him, and now this woman thinks I'm a shit mum who doesn't care. She is pretending not to care, too, but she has a plan and she is involved and she is doing it better than me.

Noah jumps in.

'We can use my colouring pens, Mummy!'

'I've got colouring pens,' says Scout.

They both look at me with pleading grins. Lo looks at me and shrugs.

'OK,' I say.

'Great,' says Lo. 'I'll bring the coloured paper, and you bring your pens, Noah. Maybe here, Tuesday week?'

'Yes!' chimes Scout.

'Sure,' I say.

She smiles, and so do I, and it looks like we have a date.

Noah is dozy as I put him to bed and give him a kiss on the forehead.

'Did you have fun?'

'Yes.'

'Do you know how much I love you?'

We stretch out our arms wide, but his move slowly.

'To Pluto and back,' he says.

'To Pluto and back,' I say.

I kiss him again, and stroke his hair.

'Thanks, Mummy.'

'What for?'

'For letting me have a playdate.'

'That's OK.'

'Can we go back tomorrow?'

'No, but we can go soon.'

He nods gently and his eyes are closing before I turn off the light.

I get to the living room and tip out his school bag. There's a book called *Reception English, Targeted Practice: Phonics*, which I've never seen before, and all scrunched up at the bottom are a little pile of notes. But what use are notes when email exists? Who runs home to strip-search a four-year-old in search of vital educational information?

There's a harvest project, there's a trip to a farm coming up, there was a photographer in, and a note from this week has a little code for the picture.

I open up my laptop and go to the website and put in the password for Noah's pictures.

And there he is: hair sticking up at the back, big smile on his face. A first moment in his new world, captured forever, with a watermark for 'Howley Photographic' stamped across his face.

He looks so perfect.

What mum wouldn't want this?

What kind of terrible mum wouldn't want this picture of her boy?

I sit for a moment, looking at his face. I told Lo I was a writer, so maybe I am, and maybe I can write about this.

One Day Soon
21:37, 19 September

The School Photo

I know what my boy looks like.

I know every curve of his face. The way his mouth is slightly uneven and how I can never get his fringe quite right.

How his eyes are so blue you feel like you're on holiday whenever you look at them.

How his bright red lips always make him look like he's just had a cherry Slurpee.

I know these things well because I see his face every day. I watch it as he eats, and as we play on the floor, and while he sits in front of the TV.

I watch him so closely that some days he turns to me and says,

'What, Mummy?' like he can feel my eyes on him.

And then school sends a little form, asking if I want a picture.

Would I like, as a minimum, to spend £10 on a mounted 7' x 5' photo of that face?

Or perhaps, 'Package 4', with eight images in varying sizes for just £45?

Here's a little example of how it would look. We've put a watermark across his face, so you can't steal it.

He may be yours, but this picture is not.

And let's not forget harvest festival, with donations collected at the school office. Please bring tinned items for those in need.

But I'm in need.

And I don't have tins for me.

13
LO

I'm perched on the edge of a kitchen chair, editing the Etisk video. It's Scout pretending to be a reporter and jumbling up questions about sustainable fashion. A mother-daughter Q&A, which I'm already slightly regretting, but has now been approved by the client. The house looks like someone's ransacked it, but Scout is asleep and I've nearly finished my work.

Dylan warmed up a bit in the end, I think. Women always hate me at first, and it matters to prove them wrong. And behind her frostiness there's warmth. I don't know if we'll be mates, but our kids are, so we'll have to make it work.

Kiddie cups and tea mugs from her visit are on the table, alongside flecks of green sludge from Scout's pesto-pasta dinner. I add the last line to the subtitles, export and send it to Jenn. I exhale loudly. It's a moment of peace, with no one needing anything, just the steady drip of the kitchen tap.

The door slams loudly and I wince, hoping Scout doesn't wake. Johno strides in, taking up space. He has a beanie on and shakes rainwater off his navy mac. He's carrying shopping bags that leave a small trail of water from the front door to the kitchen counter.

'Hey.'

'Hi. Sorry I'm late.'

As he enters the kitchen, he purses his lips, waiting for me to kiss him, so I do. A dab of skin together.

When we were in our old flat, before Scout came along, one of us returning home would mean a proper kiss. He would grab my arse and pull me to him, or I would throw myself around his neck, each of us giving the other a dramatic show of affection. It was a mini-play we performed, a deliberate exaggeration, each of us knowing their part like we were long-lost sweethearts in a 1950s matinee.

Then Scout arrived, and our welcomes deflated to a peck, like old-time marrieds in a sitcom. It was gradual, like the erosion of a riverbank or the melting of the ice caps.

His clothes smell of evening air and cigarettes, even though he doesn't smoke.

'You stink of fags.'

'Yeah, just went for a quick drink and all the cool kids were smoking.'

'So you did, too?'

'No, but they were all chatting outside. Before it rained.'

He spends more of his waking time with these people than with us and I don't really know who 'they' are.

His smell reminds me of nights that could lead anywhere. Of drinks after work and the scent of beer and fags and freedom. The smell of his aftershave as I leaned in to tell him something that would make him squeeze my knee. I can't remember the last time I went for a quick anything, other than a wee. Everything requires military planning since Scout came along.

Cut crusts from sandwiches.

Post 'uplifting' life moment.

Put shoes on feet.

Post empathetic, sad moment.

Fill in forms.

Post ad for ethical leisurewear.

But not for Johno, perhaps. Other than leaving the office a bit earlier some days for pick-up, his life has only had to slightly bend to Scout, whereas mine was bulldozed to the ground and I'm stood here staring at the rubble, wanting it to all go away while wishing it to last forever. A mother's paradox.

'So was it fun?'

'Fine,' he replies.

That's all I tend to get on the ten hours we spend apart. It's like asking Scout about her day and getting four words in response. But she's four and he's thirty-six. I've had a couple of varying responses over the last few years. 'Nothing to report, really,' is the usual go-to. Occasionally I get a gentle sigh and 'Same, same.' Sometimes he embellishes things by telling me about his lunchtime sandwich.

'What do you want for dinner?'

He unpacks with a flourish, slapping down food like a hunter returning from the field. He has five of his stock items: fishcakes, broccoli, bread, milk and a packet of chocolate digestives.

'I'll have what you're having,' I say.

'But what do you fancy?'

'I really don't mind.'

The length of the day is settling on me, and I'd like him to make this decision. He knows my dietary requirements – 'no coriander' is fairly easy to log – and we've only got fishcakes, so options are limited.

I go to the fridge and stare in there for something. There's half a bottle of corner-shop rosé with a globule of hardened ketchup on its neck.

'Fancy some wine?'

'Just a dribble,' he says, with a holiness like he's just been anointed.

I pour what's left of the bottle into two big glass goblets and walk past him to the kitchen table. Then I lick my index finger and plunge it into the salty remnants of the crisp bowl while flicking from Instagram to Influenza with the other hand.

@Mother_minded's thread has another 456 comments, mine has none. I reread Chumley_corner's comment: *Like her*.

'Scout had a playdate,' I say to Johno.

I put my phone down, the screen reflecting my silhouette, and take a sip of wine.

He hasn't asked me how my day was. He used to. He used to look at me like I was doing a poignant spoken-word performance every time I told him about my activities. Now he looks at me like I'm eating into time that could be given to his phone, or the TV, or, as currently, the *Haringey Gazette*, sitting on the counter as he peers at a photo of a man in hi-vis. A stranger in safety wear is more engaging that me. Strangers on the internet care more about my day than the man in my life.

I keep staring at my reflection in my phone, waiting for him to say something. Maybe he hasn't heard me.

'Scout had a playdate,' I say in a barbed tone and he looks up from the paper like a startled rabbit.

'Who was it with?'

'A boy in her class called Noah.'

I say this like he should know, and dislike myself for it. I take a sip of wine and turn back to my phone.

'His mum is called Dyl,' I add. 'Skinny woman, blonde, cropped hair. Not sure if you've seen her at school?'

I wonder if he'd find Dyl attractive. She has the sort of body that makes an old hoodie look good. She's tight. Firm. She looks like she's light but her body is strong. Like one of those lithe girls in pornos that gets done by a man built like The Incredible Hulk. I'm a size 14 to her 8. Stood next to her, I feel pillowy. If we hugged, I'd engulf her.

'Yeah, I met her. She looks quite knackered. She was a bit jumpy.'

He only says negative things about women he finds attractive. Or who he is worried that I might think he finds attractive.

'I don't know what she makes of me,' I say, 'but Noah and Scout seem to be best mates already.'

I might not be able to give Scout a sibling, but I can give her friends.

'Noah was born at Haringey too. They're a week apart. We must have come in as she left.'

The wine is melting away the day, making me feel lighter. I look at Johno, wondering if he remembers those first moments of Scout's life like I do. The faint smell of her head, the moment she clamped onto my nipple, connecting us with an unbreakable bond. We never really talked about her birth because there wasn't the time. Time evaporated when Scout was born.

'Do you remember that guy who started whingeing about how uncomfortable the chair was while his partner was contracting?'

'Yes,' he says, smiling. 'And that woman with eight kids, giving birth in the waiting room.'

The fishcakes are in the oven and he's chopping broccoli florets.

'Her mum just kept shouting, "She doesn't usually swear!" There's a baby clawing its way out of your daughter's vagina, love. She can swear.'

We laugh lightly, the tension evaporating slightly. I pour the rest of the wine into my mouth, hold it there like a seasoned sommelier and open my throat, like a dam releasing water. I go to the fridge and open another bottle, mesmerised by the rhythmic glug of liquid escaping into the glass.

Johno leaves his plate on the side, just inches from the dish-washer, and says, 'I'll do that later,' which seems unlikely. He reaches into the tumble dryer, feels the clothes, puts another cycle on and strolls through to the living room. My phone is on eight per cent battery, so I plug it in by the kettle while I scrape the remnants of a fishcake into the bin. As the dryer gets up to speed, I can hear him flicking between TV channels and I stand alone, enjoying the stillness. I think it's the first time I've stood still all day. I look at the time: 8.43 p.m. I imagine a nation of parents exhaling on the sofa, ready to stare at the TV while flicking to their phones. A captive audience.

'What do you want to watch?' Johno calls from the other room.

'I don't mind, you choose something.'

Anything will do. Staring at *Songs of Praise* would be a welcome distraction.

A message from Jenn cuts through the screen to remind me to post an ad tonight. It's for Picture This, a company that turns your photos into an album. My head feels full, like there's a meniscus about to overflow. I swipe to Instagram and a flood of new followers and red hearts lifts me up. I flick back to Influenza, and a new comment on @Mother_minded's post pops up.

Motherscare says: Just been BLOCKED! I simply asked if the £1,500 dress she was wearing was an advert.

I flick to the draft Picture This ad. It's an old photo of me in hospital with Scout. Johno took it, when she was barely minutes old. She's cradled in the nook of my arm, a creature so small she's barely a person. So perfect and delicate and in need of me. On my bedside table there's a book: *Dis Mem Ber* by Joyce Carol Oates. Slightly dark tales for a new mum. How naïve I was to think I'd be able to read. I breathe in and post.

> One for the memory bank? Or one for a @Picture_This! photo album? Keep your memories safe with this 24-hour photo service that can transform all your online photos into something to keep forever #makingmemories #ad.

Johno calls from the living room.

'You coming, Lo?'

'Yeah, one minute.'

I wonder what he really thinks of what I do. If it's naff or embarrassing or a means to an end. He's never stopped me, but he's never cheered me on, either. Other than when the money lands.

He's got the TV on but is plugged into his phone like it's a pacifier, soothed by a world of sports reports and obscure memes. My ad has only got twenty-seven likes and one comment so far. My mood sinks as I keep refreshing the screen, willing people to like it.

My thumb just glides over, top to bottom, top to bottom. It feels smooth against the skin, as long as I avoid the crack in the corner. I can feel my fingerprints slip gently down each time, a pause of expectation, the turn of the grey wheel while the world stops for a microsecond, and finally the reveal. One more heart, one comment. Glide. Three more hearts. Glide.

My feet feel cold on the kitchen floor and my urethra burns slightly, but I don't want to walk through the lounge and remind Johno I'm here. So I stand still, leaning against the kitchen top, absorbed by the glow.

@j&nesailing

Is nothing sacred to you? How about protecting the memories of your family from strangers on the internet?

@teats\\and//tantrums

Didn't think it would be long before the trolls came out. Ignore them LO!

My chest tightens, I breathe in. I can't ignore it, because maybe she has a point, and if I don't say something, then maybe others will join in.

'Lo, are you coming?'

His voice is a background noise as my thumbs hover above the screen. Then he uses the voice he has for Scout when she's refusing to brush her teeth.

'Do you need me to take your phone off you?'

'I'm working, Johno. Just give me a minute.'

My tone is a little snappy and he's silent. The dryer trundles around louder and I punch the pause button with my index finger.

@j&nesailing @teats\\and//tantrums

It's a valid point, so I don't think anyone is trolling exactly, but I appreciate the support. I have many memories that I don't share here; this is a snapshot of my life, if you will. But I can't make apologies for trying to carve out a career after being pushed out of the workforce. And, yes, sometimes that will involve an ad. And, yes, sometimes that involves my family. With their consent.

I refresh my screen and three people have 'liked' the comment by @j&nesailing, with twelve for @teats\\and//tantrums. The dryer door clicks, indicating it's ready to be opened. An iCal reminder flashes up on my phone. I have to fill in the school consent form for a trip to a farm.

'Lo, you coming?'

I put my phone in my pocket, gently buzzing against my thigh, and go and sit next to Johno. He's chosen a documentary on female mass-murderers. The woman on the screen looks like our dentist and I try to remember when Scout last had her teeth checked.

I creep upstairs into the bedroom to slip into my cotton nightie, trying not to disturb him. The room is dark and he's sleeping.

Light from the street lamp outside our house creeps through the gaps in the shutters like prison bars. I edge into my side, careful not to brush his leg. His body is leaden and he's breathing deeply as I stare at him, wondering what he's dreaming. His cold foot slides a little further over to my side, a sharp toenail catching my ankle. I squeeze his arm but try to end the contact.

'Night, then,' he says.

'Night, night,' I say, the second 'night' now automatic, almost parental.

We lie in silence, listening to the distant hum of the North Circular and a moped whizzing up our street like a bluebottle fly.

The day replays in my mind as I stare at the shadows of dancing trees as the wind blows outside. My ad has only 234 likes and fourteen comments, two of them negative and from anonymous accounts.

Then Johno's mass of hair and stomach inches closer to me, his erection nudging my buttocks, like a dog's nose to an owner's lap.

What signs can I possibly have given him?

He starts kissing the back of my neck and my hairs go on edge because I can't turn it on like he can.

But I also know that we will both be kinder tomorrow if we do it tonight. And we want a baby.

His hand gently moves my nightie up so our bare skin touches and I can feel him working his way over my stomach, flopped to one side like a water balloon. I feel nothing because I have everything on my mind.

Scout's consent form.

Yoghurts for packed lunch box.

Kitchen tap drip.

Reply to Amara.

Book smear test.

My mind whirrs as I roll over and kiss him. Our teeth clash slightly, but it doesn't deter him. I wonder if he's thinking of the last YouPorn star he wanked to, or of someone else. Eilis, perhaps, or Dyl with her nipples pushing through that white top.

I lean in and we kiss aggressively. It's a frenzied exchange to save us having to be tender. We paw at each other and I slowly want this, a feeling in the real world, so I pull him close and he pushes inside me. Our pubic hair rubs together like two Brillo pads, and there's a rhythmic clap of untoned bodies colliding.

Then there's a loud creak outside the door.

We both stop, holding our breath and each other in the darkness, wondering if Scout is there. He withdraws and leans over to open the bedroom door a crack, like an ageing contortionist.

'It's just the bathroom blind in the wind,' he whispers, closing our door again.

He looks at me, and I half expect him to say, 'where were we?'

14

DYLAN

It's nearly 1.00 a.m., I'm smoking out of the window and I should sleep, but I can't. I check my phone and exactly eight people have seen my school-photo post.

The thing with a blog is, I don't know who they are or how they got there. They were probably just searching for photographers, not for me griping.

All this fucking earache.

I breathe out, think about the day. Johno and Lo won't be sneaking rollies out the window and tapping out crappy blog posts.

I expect she made food, as Johno tucked up Scout and read her stories about princesses that slay dragons.

Or maybe he cooks.

Maybe he came back with nice red wine and fresh ingredients, gave Lo a kiss as he walked through the door, then laid things out on the countertop because he likes to make food for her while music plays.

Maybe they still flirt a bit while they tell each other about their days and she told him about me.

Maybe he left a sauce bubbling in the pan and they put their hands on each other and he lifted her onto the kitchen counter and they let the food burn because he hadn't seen her all day. Maybe she wrapped her legs around him, because they need each other so much, and they had sex right there on the marble counter, and afterwards they laughed about how the sauce has burned dry, but they didn't care, they just dabbed at it with crusty bread and it still tasted good as they drank their wine.

Maybe that's what they did, and then they went to bed.

And I wonder what their bedroom looks like, so I pick up my phone and turn to Instagram and have a look.

A few pictures back, Lo is perched on the end of the bed, taking a picture of herself in the bedroom mirror, looking stern and meaningful. The room is neat, stylish. The walls are pale green and the duvet cover is a fresh baby blue. You can see some laundry piled in the corner, for authenticity.

When you show someone your bed, you're inviting them to think about you in it. You're making them picture your warm body beneath the sheets, and making them wonder what you wear. Is it thin and delicate and silk, or do you wrap up like an old maid and top it off with woollen socks? Maybe they wear nothing, and let the duvet just rest on their skin.

I skim on, through their beautiful home. She is on her green velvet sofa with its thick, soft cushions, sipping coffee on a Sunday morning. And then, a few posts earlier, Johno's lying in the same space, as Scout jumps on top of him, caught in mid-flight, about to land on her dad. Then Lo's in the kitchen, acting all confused about how to make a cake. Theirs is a warm space with full cupboards and soft edges, and for just a little while I was there.

I went to give Noah a friend, but all I've done is show him what he doesn't have.

This flat is the best place we've ever lived, and now it feels like nothing.

But this place is a miracle, because when I met JD I was seventeen and staying in the box room of a cheap rental, with my mattress and sheets on a painted wooden floor, living with strangers and working in a café.

And one night, in a crappy old boozer, I met this thirty-year-old guy with grey-brown hair and a smile that stole the room and he came back and stayed for a week. We slept and ate and drank and when we woke up hung-over, we would roll into each other to make ourselves feel better.

And that was him in my life.

A month later, he took me to the Savoy in a black cab. I was in trainers and jeans and looked like a busker, and he ordered champagne and caviar and steak and said to bring it all at once. And when it came, he spread the little eggs all over the meat like jam and laughed at the waiter's face.

When he was done, he dropped £400 in the middle of the table and gave me his grin.

See me in the gents.

And after that we got a night bus home, all the way to that big old forgotten-about house in Woolwich, and it was the last place I lived without him. I lived there with three guys, and JD didn't really like that.

One was Jordi, who grew mint and spuds in the garden and drank tea and smoked spliffs and played guitar sitting on the landing windowsill.

Until one day Jordi was on the patio and there were these sounds from a splintering guitar and Jordi had his shin sticking out.

Careful, Jordi.

And all I could think was, 'But he's already fallen, JD.'

And then we had to leave, because of that accident.

So this place is a miracle.

It's nothing like hers, but it's a miracle for me.

One Day Soon
01:27, 20 September

<u>The Woman At the Spyhole</u>

We moved about.

Hostels for a bit, if we had to. Flats sometimes, if they were cheap. I worked in cafés and bars; he did things he shouldn't.

One place had a spyhole in the door.

It had a little brass cover and made everything outside curve at the edges. A little thing for peeping at the postman or the woman opposite. Her door was painted the same charcoal grey, because aspirational living only counts if everyone does it the same, and the grey matched her suit the first time we smiled on the stairs.

'Hi!'

'Hey!'

Now that's enough for a London neighbour.

No need to stop, and we don't stay in one place long.

And then one night, he pushed me out there onto the landing.

'Fuck off, then.'

And a slam, and me on the concrete in just a white T-shirt and knickers.

'What are you doing? It's cold out here!'

But he just turned up the telly for some game with a roaring crowd.

'I'm sorry.'

He ignored me, so I said it louder.

'I'm sorry!'

And I heard her little brass cover, just as he came back out. A little scratch over the eyehole, as he grabbed my arm.

'Shut up and get inside.'

And a little cuff round the back of the head.

After that, she didn't smile any more on the stairs. Just little nods, until we moved on.

But she could have said.

She could have touched my arm and said, 'That's not OK.'

Because no one else saw the things he did, except the woman at the peephole.

And I stayed with him for five years.

And he's still in my head every day.

15

OCTOBER

LO

The Tube rattles and shakes its heavy load of commuters, but I have a seat, so feel like one of the lucky ones. And the huddled bodies are a chance to watch people. Opposite me is a woman eating a chopped-up apple out of a small Tupperware box, who has lots of empty piercings in her ears and nose, like divots from a former life.

I'm meeting Jenn at The Artemis, a women-only club. They're breaking down barriers for any woman who can afford the two-grand membership fee. It's set in a beautiful Georgian town house right between Hyde Park and Green Park, and you can apparently see the Serpentine from the rooftop bar.

I'm wearing brogues and cut-off red trousers with a loose cashmere jumper. My ankles are chilly, but I look like I've made an effort without seeking attention.

Drop-off was good today. Scout brought her uniform into us in the bedroom and said she was ready to go to school, even though it was barely light. When we got to the gate, she practically sprinted in, leaving me behind. It stings a bit, to see this tiny part of you existing independently, but it is a warm sting.

She is creating her own world, in the tiniest of ways, making friends and discovering leaf rubbings.

The Tube gets to Green Park and I march up the escalator until the autumn air hits my face. I get my phone out, type in the address and start following the blue dotted line on Google Maps. The day is crisp and bright and ready, and the low sun throws long shadows from the grand facades. London sometimes feels like it's pushing you down, a grimy duvet weighing you to the pavement, and then there's a day like today, when the clouds dissolve and you look up at the rooftops, each one different to the last, glass new-builds by stately Georgians.

These are the days that make me feel like it's working. That I may be 'selling my family on the internet', as one follower called it, but I can also be with them when I want. It's about choice. Working and parenting is one of the biggest conflicts I've experienced. Everything in me wants to be with her, but whatever job I do, someone else needs me to turn up, to show up, to lean in. And I don't have an option not to work, so for now this is it. Today, at least, I don't feel redundant.

The Artemis has a plain green door and shuttered ground-floor windows. There's an old newsagent to the left and a Japano-Chilean fusion café to the right. By the Artemis door is a tiny buzzer with a camera above. I ring and a dislocated voice answers.

'Hello?'

'Hello. I'm Lois Knox. I have a meeting.'

She says no more and I hear a buzz and a metallic clack and push the heavy door open to step in and inhale the perfumed air. In front of me is an oak-panelled reception desk, with a pink neon 'Women supporting women' sign above two of the most beautiful females I've ever seen. One has very straight fair hair swept around to tumble down her right shoulder, the other has dark hair, pulled back in a ponytail to form the faintest border to her skull. They both have shimmering white blouses that hang perfectly off delicate shoulders. The blonde one smiles, while the ponytail looks back to her keyboard.

'Hello. Who is your meeting with?'

'Jenn Riley.'

'Are you a member, Lois?'

'No.'

She smiles again.

'Please take a seat in the lounge, and someone will take you to your host.'

She points to my left and a collection of chaises longues, armchairs and sofas, each in a different shade of pastel. The carpet is a monochrome houndstooth and there are beautiful redwood coffee tables. There's an oil painting of a dog with a goose's head staring down from the fireplace.

I flick to my phone: my latest post is going well. It's just a video of me on a little rant about phonics and asking when the letter C became a 'curly kuh'. Seems many others feel my pain.

I tap my search bar, add an 'I' and autofill knows what's next. I'm back on Influenza, gliding through to @Mother_minded's thread. It feels like a dirty little secret, but one that 37,178 people are 'viewing' with me. The comments are slowing and I open to the most recent.

Getoffmyinternetnow says: It's taken me a while, but I've done some digging (I knew my accountancy training would come in handy eventually) and found her Companies House returns. She got a firm called Mind-Full Ltd (very naff) in her husband's name.

Last year's turnover was £672,000. AFTER dividends! See for yourselves! I guess depression can be more profitable than people think.

She's added screen grabs from the Companies House website.

A waitress interrupts my scrolling.

'Lois?'

'Yes!'

I say it a bit too loudly, almost a shout, and I feel the receptionists' eyes glance over.

'This way please.'

The waitress smiles and walks ahead. She has the same shimmering blouse, and is wearing slim-fit black trousers.

In the restaurant, Jenn sits at a table for two, beside a wall papered to look like a forest. She's in a sheened, black 80s-cut power suit and white trainers. When she sees me, she leaps to her feet and hugs me like a long-lost relative.

'All right, love, how are you?'

She can only be in her mid-twenties, but the way she says 'love' – with just a lingering hint of her Brummie accent – makes me feel like she's a tender auntie.

'Good, yes, this is nice, isn't it?'

'I know, lovely, right?'

'And your hair is amazing.'

Her jet-black locks have been sculpted into fat curls flying out across her head. She's mesmeric, and I spend half a second just staring at her and remembering what it is to be that box-fresh.

'I call it my Medusa look. One glance at me and you turn to stone.'

The waitress pours us water from a jug on the table and steps away as we sit.

'How long have you been a member?'

'Since it opened,' she says. 'I know someone on the launch team. I could nominate you, if you want? They need to fill it up.'

She lifts up the menu and peers down, so I do the same. On the back of her menu is an arrow motif, repeated in miniature on the inside pages of mine.

Our table is set with forks that look like tiny tridents, and at the end of the dining room is a two-metre-high classical portrait of a woman in a field, her hand reaching to a quiver of arrows on her back. Her hair is plaited in dark bunches either side of her head, and her soft white dress is almost transparent, falling perfectly over every curve of her full hips and breasts.

'What's with the arrows?'

'Artemis is Goddess of the Hunt.'

She says this casually, as though it should be known.

'Oh, I see.'

'It's in the brochure. We didn't do much classics in my school either. Now are you eating, love?'

As she says this, a waiter appears at our table. He is beautiful. Not just handsome, but stop-and-stare beautiful. Like his jaw has been carved in marble. He has a perfectly flat stomach and I can't help picturing a light six-pack beneath his shirt, its thick white cotton tucked neatly into black trousers.

'Are you ready to order?'

He holds his pad and pen and I'm transfixed by the bend of his arms. The shirt bunches just below rounded biceps.

'Maybe a minute more?'

He smiles at Jenn and steps away. We exchange a look.

'I know,' she says. 'That's Arno.'

'I'd have that on toast.'

'Ha! But don't you think he's a bit too . . .'

'Sculpted?'

'Yeah.'

'No, I do not.'

I look at the menu and I'm suddenly very hungry.

'I thought it was women only, though?'

'They allow male staff.'

'So you can't have a meeting with a man?'

'In a world of patriarchal absolutism, a space for the female to flower, the matriarch to rise, for women to support women.'

'Oh.'

'That was in the brochure, too.'

Our food arrives: an egg-white omelette for Jenn, smashed avocado and scrambled eggs for me, with a side of toast.

Arno lays down the food like it's delicate silk and I say 'thank you' too much. As we begin to eat, Jenn turns to business.

'Now: there are a couple of reasons I wanted to meet here. Mostly, this is a celebration.'

She dramatically hoists up a bottle of Veuve Clicquot from under the table. It's a 2008 vintage. Whenever there was cause for celebration at Darby Cooper, there would be an uncomfortable gathering of colleagues around your desk as you blew out a solitary candle on a Colin the Caterpillar cake, everyone clapping like seals. One of the paralegals once signed my birthday card, 'sorry you're leaving'. This ritual was repeated for baby showers, leaving dos and engagements, Colin always appearing centre-stage like a nativity donkey.

'That's for smashing past 50,000 followers. Well done.'

'Oh, wow, thank you.'

Jenn is the closest thing I have to a colleague, and for the first time since Scout was cut out of me, I feel needed by someone that doesn't want their bottom wiped. She has a roster of ten 'talents', and I'm the smallest, but this feels like the first time I might have proved to her that I can do this.

'You've earned it, love. Now even more exciting, if that's possible. Some new jobs. First, the insurance firm, Allegiance, would like you to speak on a panel for them. They like what you're doing for breastfeeding and it's well paid. That's all signed off.'

'Amazing!'

'But that's not the biggie. You know WeAreFemForm?'

'The sanitary pads?'

'They want you in an ad. On TV.'

As she says this, her eyes widen and her voice rises up a little. The tiny row of diamond studs in her ears reflects the light from the chandelier.

'What?'

'Primetime: ITV, Sky, Channel 4, the lot.'

'What?'

'You heard me: it's twelve grand for the shoot day and usage. More if it runs longer than a year.'

'What?'

'Will you stop saying, "what" and say, "thanks, Jenn!"'

'Thanks, Jenn!'

That's five months of my previous salary. In one day. How many dreary press releases would I have to write to make that up? I'd sell anything for that return.

'This is big, love. They've got you and eight others, and it's not just the money. This is profile: national telly, great visibility. People will see your face right in the middle of Corrie.'

'STOP! Me and Deirdre Barlow, together at last.'

'She's not in it anymore, but yes, you'll be landing in the homes of the nation. Talking about periods, but still, the female body is dead on-brand for you.'

My arms go a little light and I sit back in my chair, resting them either side of my plate. I'm too excited to eat. This means I'll be able to spend more time with Scout. Maybe I can afford to put my phone down for a bit.

'Seriously, Jenn, thank you. When I started, I really didn't think anything could come of this.'

'Well, it's all down to you. You've got something people like.'

'Ha! Well, that's a first.'

She smiles at me, takes a trident-fork full of omelette and sips at her black coffee while it all sinks in. I exhale a little.

'Maybe I actually can afford membership here.'

'You definitely can. Arno's not included, though. But look, I said it was "mostly" a celebration.'

'Oh, yes.'

I hold onto the neck of the champagne bottle, feeling like she's about to take something back.

'Well, your following is still rising, but your engagement's falling. Not enough people are liking your posts.'

'Oh.'

'It happens, we've seen it before, just not normally this early. You normally see it around 200k.'

'Oh. What does it mean?'

'You need to post more. Feed the beast. The algorithm rewards volume. The more you post, the more new people it will serve your content to.'

'But I post every day.'

'Try twice a day. Do more stories. Get more personal, show them who you really are, what your life is like. People love peeking through the keyhole, so why not fling open the door?'

A stab of adrenaline hits my chest and a little surge runs through my heart. What more is there to say?

*

Arno takes our plates, and Jenn calls for the bill. I've barely touched my food since she mentioned the ad.

'What will I have to do for WeAreFemForm?'

'Turn up, look pretty, be yourself. You'll ace it.'

'OK.'

'There will be briefs, don't worry.'

She punches in her pin like it's a code to a secret-service HQ as Arno looks away.

'Now,' she says, 'I've got to get back, but lovely to see you.'

'OK, can I stay and work?'

'Sure, soak it up. Enjoy the view.'

She gives me a knowing look as she stands and we hug, while Arno slips away.

'Take care, love, we're proud of you. Now get that post frequency up.'

She walks out and I settle back down.

I flick to my phone. I need to get the screen fixed, before that crack spreads. Four new followers, seventy-two likes, eight messages.

The messages are mounting and I need to clear them. Mostly they're nice: laugh emojis, women saying they've experienced things I've written about. Each one gives me a little glow, like a gentle pat on the back or a squeeze on the arm. When you work in an office, you never really get praise. A casual 'great, thanks' that means nothing. Every appraisal meeting with a manager has to have strengths and weaknesses, evenly balanced, to keep you on your toes. In the spring before I left, I got Darby Cooper more positive press coverage than they'd ever had in one quarter. After telling me how impressed they were, my boss reminded me that my grammar could be sloppy: 'We're also judged on our internal comms,' he said. 'And people here care about apostrophes.'

On those rare occasions I got a heartfelt 'well done', I floated about the place for days, convinced I'd one day be CEO. Until someone would knock a press release I'd written, not wanting me to get above my station.

But now I get those little highs every day. Little boosts, little digital high-fives. Little fleeting gifts of praise from thousands of women across the country and beyond.

So I scroll through, and I read them all. Each one sparks a tiny glow, a micro-smile, a wisp of appreciation. I am doing well. I am earning money and making change.

But I have to read on for the other messages, too. The women in mourning for lives that didn't form, the women whose careers ended because they managed to breed, the ones who want to leave their husband, the ones with a cause. They can't be left to linger as 'seen' among the thousands of fist-bumps and cry-laughs. Once you've 'seen' someone, you can't just turn on your heel and pretend they're not there. I don't want to make anyone feel as small as I did.

'Hello.'

I look up and it's Arno. His eyes are a remarkably deep brown and it feels like he's looking right into me.

'Hi,' I smile.

'Could I take your name?'

'Lo. Lo Knox.'

I find myself folding my hands over each other.

'And are you a member here?'

'No.'

'Oh . . .'

Arno looks disappointed in me.

134

'. . . It's just, I'm very sorry, but guests can only stay with a host.'

He looks upon me sadly, like I've ordered the finest champagne but had my card declined.

'But my friend said it would be OK. I was going to do some work.' My voice is a little pleading, and Arno sadly tilts his beautiful face.

'I'm so sorry, madam. Do you have anything in the cloakroom?'

I walk down the street, feeling like I've been through a very polite eviction. I need to find a quiet spot to work. Piccadilly has too much traffic, and a chain café will have too much background noise.

But these are the London streets I love. Grand Georgian homes with giant greystone fronts and black cast-iron railings. You can't help but imagine where you might have fitted when these places were built: dabbed in powder and wig, draped over a chaise longue, or scrabbling below stairs, hoping not to catch the master's temper?

In a Georgian garden square, I find a little bench and take my perch. There are giant oaks and elms all around the perimeter, with dappled autumn sun picking its way through. It seeps in, like yellow and orange ink on one of Scout's felt-tip scribble sessions. I look up at the sky and close my eyes for a moment, absorbing the light.

The air feels better, and the trees fight off the distant sounds of traffic. It might not be a members' club, but it feels good. I have got a TV ad, I am earning on my own terms, and this afternoon I will collect my daughter from school for a playdate with her new friend. I flick my phone, and skim over the private messages.

'. . . Thanks so much for all you're doing . . .'

'. . . Where can I get post-miscarriage support? . . .'

'. . . Yeah, screw you curly kuh!'

☺

☺

☺

16

DYLAN

I grin at Noah, while Lo serves the kids squash in matching green-plastic cups. We're in their kitchen again: me and the kids sat around the table so Noah and Scout can do their harvest project.

'Can't be any fights over who gets which cup if they're all the same,' Lo says.

'Yes. I do hate mismatched crockery when catering for under-fives.'

She smiles, but I'm not sure why I said that. It was meant to be funny, but I think it came out snide. Maybe she got everything to match for the kid that that won't come, and I should just be a nicer person.

'Thank you,' says Noah.

'Thanks, *Mom*,' says Scout, adopting an American accent. Both the kids laugh.

Lo looks at me, a little confused.

'Not sure where that came from.'

Lo's been at a meeting, and is dressed in this beautiful wool jumper that makes you want to stroke it. She pulls out some yellow paper from a bag and waves it in the air.

'I've gone full *Blue Peter*,' she says, and throws it on the table. 'Thanks so much for doing this, Lo.'

'Oh, it's fine.'

The kids grab at everything else as it comes: more coloured paper, this time orange and green, a glue stick, dry pasta, a new set of colouring pencils, kids' scissors. I've brought Noah's little bag of felt tips and my boy looks comfortable here. It is natural for him, to be here and to play. More natural than for me.

Her home is a bit less foreign the second time, but it is still hers. I've kept my shoes on, but still can't be sure she's happy about it. I think I know where the bog is, but I'd still ask to use it.

As the kids sift their stash, Scout does a funny face, like she has just been handed something hilarious and alien.

'What's *this* for?' she asks, holding up some macaroni.

She is a performer, playing the room for laughs.

'Well, Scouty, when I was little, we would glue macaroni to paper.'

'You would *glue it to paper*?'

She is baffled, hamming it up for the entertainment of my boy.

'Yes,' says Lo. 'I guess it is a *bit funny*.'

Lo plays along, exaggerating her voice and her expressions. They're performing, being engaged, showing each other that they are listening. Maybe this is how they always are: energised, giving each other loving attention.

We all look at the little craft centre we've created.

'Where shall we start?' I ask.

Lo has the school note to hand.

'Create a scene to show autumn harvest and all the food that farmers provide. You could paint a farm, or do drawings of the food. Let your imagination run wild.'

We stare at the equipment in front of us.

'Well,' says Lo.

'The yellow can be bananas,' says Scout.

'Yes, although bananas don't really grow in England,' says Lo.

Noah chips in.

'Can I make the farm?'

Lo looks to Scout for any objections.

'Great idea, Noah. How about you make the farm picture, and Scout can make the food picture? The macaroni could be wheat in the field. And, Scouty, you could draw food on different coloured bits of paper, then cut them out and stick them on a new piece.'

And so we go to work. Scout begins to scribble away with her pencils, while I help Noah to dab glue over dried macaroni. Lo looks at me a little conspiratorially, like we've nailed this.

'Well great,' she says, 'I'll get the kettle on.'

We're sitting opposite each other at their table, tea in hand and our kids by our sides. Scout is drawing something that might be a marrow. Noah is drawing what looks like a farm.

While the kids work, there's a silence. These are the moments I guess were always coming. Sitting around with another mum, trying to find some connection because our kids make each other happy. I smile at her. If I can make chat with dead-eyed office managers, I can do it with her.

'How has your week been?'

'Good, great. Busy, but fun,' she says.

She is upbeat, fizzing a bit. Like she has news to share but doesn't want to show off.

'How about you?'

She fixes me with the same smile she gives to Scout.

'Good, yeah, I sold some water-cooler contracts.'

It sounds lame as I say it. Like I'm rolling my eyes to grumble about the weather. Like it's lame and I'm lame, but I'm not. I'm good at it. Probably better than she would be.

'Great. I meant to ask what you were tele-selling. People will always need water!'

'Yes, we do coffee vending machines, too.'

It sounds pathetic.

'And I've been writing,' I add.

'That's great.'

She says this politely. She thinks I'm a hobby scribbler, banging out Year Nine poetry in my bedroom.

'It's just for my blog, but a few people like it.'

She smiles again, a little faintly. I wonder if she gets this a lot: Hey, Mrs Social Media, I do words too!

'Do you want to have a look?'

I don't know why I'm pushing this. I don't know why I'm dishing up my homework to her. But I've never spoken to a living soul who's read my words, and she smiles.

'I'd love to!'

I think she means it, and for a moment a little of her fizzing is for me.

I call up the site on my phone and click through to the post about Dad's suicide.

'This was a recent one.'

She takes my phone and reads in silence and then her head rears back and her face has this amazed, sad look, like she's a lady vicar who's stumbled into a dogging hotspot.

'Dyl, this is . . .'

What: Shit? Needy? Boring?

'It's so . . . moving.'

She goes quiet, but I want to know what she's really thinking.

The kids continue to scribble.

'Dyl, it's . . . You're going to make me cry.'

When she says my name, I feel a little rush. A little tickle of pride.

'It's just a hobby, really.'

'No. It's more than that. No one else is going to shout about it if you don't, Dyl.'

She looks serious. Like it's touched her. Like a new colour has washed over her, and I've never seen my words do that. I've given her the saddest part of my life, and now she's felt it too and maybe she understands me.

'Is that . . .'

She stumbles a little, whispers so the kids can't hear.

'You were so young.'

'Yes. It was a long time ago.'

I try to sound noble as I say this. Like I am brave and stoic.

She puts her hand over mine. Just a gentle touch, like you might for a little old lady in a home, and rubs her thumb over the back of my hand. Her eyes look right into me.

I haven't told anyone about Dad for years, and I'd forgotten how it feels. You are injecting sorrow into them. Or guilt, because they haven't suffered. I see the sadness on her and I want to take it all back. I shake my head a little, want to change the subject.

'You're looking great today. Where were you?'

She raises her head, feels my shift of tone, smiles again.

'In town. I tried to work in this Mayfair club earlier, but they kicked me out.'

She smirks a little at the memory, rolls her eyes, turns back to my blog like she's rereading the post about Dad.

'Why did they kick you out?'

'Well, I'm not a member.'

'Ha!'

My laugh is a bit too sharp, a relief after the moment between us, and the kids look up from their work.

'Yeah,' she smiles too. 'Bit embarrassing . . .'

I can't imagine being someone who is so completely sure of themselves they would walk into a club where they weren't a member and just expect to belong. But I guess she just expects to belong everywhere. Clubs, school gates, Instagram.

'Can I ask you something?'

'Sure,' she says.

She lays down my phone again, looks up like she's lifting her head from the water.

'Aren't you worried about all the stuff you put online? Like you'll come home one day and find some perv at the bottom of the garden?'

'A tiny bit, but I've never really had any grief from men. One guy told me to put my "skanky bangers" away on a breastfeeding post . . .'

Scout looks up from her colouring: 'What's a skanky banger?'

'Nothing, darling,' says Lo. 'Mummy's just talking about work.'

Lo turns her head to the chair at the head of the table and moves round to it, placing herself diagonally next to me. She lowers her voice, leans a bit closer, and I get the briefest scent of a honeysuckle perfume.

'. . . But within five minutes, skanky-banger guy had a hundred women commenting and messaging and telling him to shut up and that they knew where he worked and he ran away and never came back.'

'Ooh. It's like you've got a hit squad.'

I say it as a joke, but it must be nice to have a crew. People to look out for you and take care of your enemies.

142

'Well, it's a bit more that we stand up for each other. If guys attack, it's just insults and they're mostly not even spelled properly. Maybe a creepy aubergine.'

'So you don't get anything?'

Her voice drops a bit further.

'Have you heard of Influenza?'

'What, like flu?'

'I think it's a play on "influencer", but it's a chat board. There's quite a bit on there.'

'Like what?'

She taps her phone, turns to show me a clunky chat-board website. There's text everywhere, a muddle of tags and threads and exclamation marks, and it's all a bit hard to follow.

'Some of it's reasonable,' she says. 'Like questioning what people are doing, pointing out hidden ads. Some of it's just women chatting, making friends. But there's a lot of calling women liars, and making things up, I think.'

'About you?'

'Not yet.'

She says this like someone in a chat board can magically reach through the screen and get you. And then we're interrupted.

'Why doesn't Noah have a daddy?'

Lo looks mortified. Scout is still colouring as she asks the question. Just drops it in, like she's in need of a biscuit.

'Darling, that's a bit rude,' says Lo.

'He's dead,' says Noah.

Lo goes pale. Even with the make-up, the colour has finally flushed from her face.

Noah is matter-of-fact, like he's asking to borrow another pen, because that's how I've always been with him. We are heaping tragedy upon tragedy on this woman, and this one's not even true.

'How did he die?'

Lo shouts, 'Scout, please!'

Her daughter looks up, scared and chastised, and so does Noah.

Lo softens her voice. 'Please, darling, some questions are too—'

'It was a car crash,' says Noah, 'before I was born.'

He says it plainly, and it punches my heart. A lie that can't be fixed.

Because what can I tell him?

'*Your dad pushed a Spanish guy out the window and broke his leg, Noh.*'

'*Your dad drove all my friends away and took my money, Noh.*'

'*Your dad doesn't know where we live and I want to keep it that way, Noh.*'

'*Your dad made me want to open up all those old scars on my arms, Noh.*'

The room falls silent and Lo leans over to me, puts her hand on mine. She is warm, her hand soft, she rubs her thumb over my finger, looks like tears will spill out of her.

'It's OK,' I tell her.

She looks grief-stricken, and it brings a new sting of guilt, because now she thinks I'm some widow as well as an orphan.

'It . . .' I start to speak, but then stop. I never thought about what I'd say to grown-ups, because I didn't think they'd ever be asking. Saying he's dead works for Noah, because it ends it.

But now Lo is wearing my fake grief, and my real grief for Dad, and stroking my hand like I've endured a tragedy, mourning for a man who is still alive and might even be looking for us right now.

Dumb cow.

'It's OK,' I say to her. 'We'd . . .' I drop my voice to a whisper. 'We'd separated. It had been a difficult relationship.'

She nods a little and doesn't quite know what to say, so she stares right into me.

'It's just . . .' she whispers. 'It's just so shit. You never know what someone else is going through.'

'Really, it's OK. It was all a long time ago.'

She's quiet again, and breathes out hard, and I turn to our little craft session.

'Well, this is going very well, isn't it, kids?'

'Yeah,' says Scout, with a sniff.

She has scribbled fruit-like shapes in many different colours. Noah doesn't reply. They are both entranced, happy in their work. He has drawn a wonky farm with a roof and a big smudge of what might be smoke. He has drawn a cow-like thing and given it black-and-white splotches. His imaginary field is full of macaroni wheat and he looks happy.

But my little lie grows bigger with everyone that hears it, and I wonder what little scars I am making inside him.

There's a rattle at the door and Scout's head perks up like a meerkat.

'Daddy's home!'

She jumps from her chair and sprints through the living room to wrap herself around Johno's legs before he can close the door.

'Daddy!'

It is a giant, loving squeeze. She clamps herself to him, only easing as he lifts her up and she can squeeze her arms around his neck.

'Daddy, can I be your tie?'

She hangs there, her tiny arms wrapped around his neck, and he walks through to the kitchen, speaking like a circus ringleader.

'Hello, darling! Do you like my new tie?'

Noah laughs, and Johno sees us and very gently eases Scout off like he's embarrassed. Like no one should see this softness.

'Come on now, little tie,' he says, 'back to work.'

And while this show goes on, water builds in Lo's eyes and she looks down because she can't look at me. Like her living partner is an extra torture to Widow Dyl, and for a moment I want to tell her: it's OK, it's a lie, it was just better that way. But how could she ever understand?

She looks up to Johno, whatever she's feeling sucked back in, and fixes a warm smile.

'You're early,' she says as he steps over to give her a soft kiss on the lips.

As he leans in, she holds still, making him reach, an awkward moment caught by me.

'Had a meeting in Camden,' he says. 'Closer to here than the office, so thought I'd stick it to the man and knock off early.'

He smiles, shrugs and turns his eyes to me.

'Hi, I'm Johno, we met in the playground.'

'Yes, I'm Dylan.'

'Like Bob. I remember.'

He shakes my hand again, smiles and holds his eyes on me before turning to Lo.

'What's all this about?'

'This is our harvest project,' says Lo.

'Exciting.'

His tone suggests it isn't.

'Well,' he says, 'since we've got company, maybe . . .'

He mimes drink, just above the kids' eyeline, and marches to the fridge.

'Do we want red or white? Dyl?'

'I don't really drink.'

'I can make them very small,' he says, eyes pleading a bit.

'I'll have white,' says Lo.

He pulls a new bottle from the fridge door, two glasses from a cabinet, and places them on the counter, then goes back for a third, which he waves in the air for a moment while looking at me, his eyebrows raised.

'OK, yeah, a small one.'

He joins us at the table, opposite me and diagonally next to Lo, opens the bottle with a pop, pours two large glasses and a slightly smaller one.

'Just a small for you.'

'Thanks,' I say.

'Thanks, darling,' says Lo, and we all clink.

'Here's to autumn harvest then,' says Johno, before taking a long sip.

He looks at me like he's about to ask something, but I get in first. I've talked about myself enough today.

'What's your work then?'

'I'm in the music business,' he says.

'He's an accountant,' says Lo.

'In the music business,' says Johno.

He smiles wryly at her, then more fully at me. They are teasing each other, I think. Or maybe she always does that to him.

'And what about you, Dylan?'

'Dylan's a writer,' says Lo, and just for a moment I feel myself flush.

'That's exciting,' says Johno.

'It's just for a blog,' I tell him.

'Her writing's incredible,' says Lo.

'So we're both basically artists,' he says to me. 'You're in publishing, I'm in music, we bring joy to people.'

'Well, dunno about that. People have to read it first.'

'Yeah, no one's listening to my tunes either.'

Lo laughs hard.

'Your what? Have you been secretly making *phat beats* in the cupboard under the stairs?'

He sighs a little sadly and looks straight at me.

'I'm not really making music. I never actually got past grade two on the triangle.'

I smile back.

'I don't think they do grades on the triangle.'

He shrugs.

'No. Maybe they should. It could be my entry to the arts.'

'Talking of which,' says Lo, 'there was one very exciting thing today.' She stands, reclaims the attention of the room, and walks over to the family corkboard. 'These came.'

She pulls out four long paper tickets in a lairy blue with gold foil.

'What is it?' asks Scout.

'Well . . .'

She passes one to me. Across the front are three dancers in mid-leap, two women and a man, and each of them in body stockings and insect costumes. The man is a beetle, one woman a butterfly, the other some kind of lizard. Across the centre in gold foil is the word 'Savannah!' and below that, 'The Premiere'. It's dated for Saturday.

'What is it, Mummy?'

'Well, Scouty, it's a special kind of show where dancers dress up like bugs and animals.'

'Oh.'

She's not quite sure how to process this, so Lo has another go.

'It's a circus, but with people.'

'A circus?'

This lands better, and Noah is interested now, too.

'Can Noah come?'

'Well,' Lo looks at me, 'I've got four tickets . . .'

'How much are they?'

'They're free.'

Of course. Lo looks at me a little longer.

'What do you think?'

She is beaming. Smiling straight at me like she's about to burst. She's trying to hide it, but I think she's almost as excited as Scout. Maybe she thinks this will cheer me up. I'd feel like I was suffocating a seal if I said no.

'Is Scout going?' asks Noah.

'Of course,' says Lo. 'I wouldn't leave little Scouty behind, would I?'

She leans down to give her daughter a squeeze, which she resists, but not very hard.

And that's it. It's agreed.

The four of us are off to the circus.

17
LO

There's a woman on the door giving away small butterfly balloons on sticks. She's wearing a sleeveless dress in an African print, even though it's nine degrees and we can see our breath in the mid-afternoon light as we queue. She smiles at us, eyes not matching her grin, and I take two balloons for Noah and Scout and walk into the theatre foyer, hot air from the overhead heaters acting like an invisible door.

'Can we keep these?'

Noah looks up at Dyl.

'I guess so,' Dyl says.

'Yes, you can keep them,' says Scout.

'Wow. That's kind of them,' I tell her.

I want Scout to know that getting things for your mere presence isn't normal. I also quite want Dyl to know that I realise this and am impressing it on my child.

There's a neat row of hundreds of yellow and blue goody bags lining the wall beneath the box office, which isn't in use because everyone already has a ticket. A woman in a leopard-print coat peers into one of the bags, clasping a plastic champagne flute in one hand and a boy with his face painted like a tiger in the other. She steps away, a little like a leopard herself, having sniffed the carrion and decided it will keep for later.

Dyl's fingers are wrapped around Noah's tiny hand. She's wearing dark brown lipstick, and as she walks, she pins her sleeves over her wrists with her fingers.

A giddy press officer in a pink suit and patent brogues approaches with a clipboard and ushers us towards the velvet-roped photo wall. Dyl steps back with Noah as we move onto the red carpet, which is more of a rug and looks like it could be a sample from Flooring Warehouse. Two bored photographers are poised as the PR shouts to them, 'Lo Knox, The Lo Down,' which they scribble into their notepads. I have no idea where the photo is going to be published – or who would be interested – but this is the tap dance we have to do to secure lukewarm Prosecco and tickets to an insect musical.

The camera flashes fire off and Scout and I stand centre-stage, blinded by the lights. Scout blinks up at me and whispers:

'Were those present bags for us?'

'Maybe. If you're good.'

Another PR raises her eyes at me. 'Thank you sooo much,' she says.

She points her arm westward like a weathervane, indicating it's time to get out of the way. Dyl and Noah have been ushered behind the photographers, and we head up the gold-railed staircase to the main circle.

Along the aisles, attractive boys with white gloves offer up tiny maggot pancakes like they're ice creams. There seem to be edible bugs in all the food, but no one is eating because cricket tempura is not very family-friendly.

'I'm hungry, can I have a snack?' says Scout.

'Me, too,' says Noah.

I take a blini and pick off the maggots, placing them in a napkin like they're about to be embalmed. I squat down and offer one to Scout, who scrunches up her face in disgust.

'You left its head. There's a head on it.'

Noah is breathing heavily over my shoulder like the insect might spring back to life and he needs me as his armour. Dyl looks down at us.

'No I didn't, look,' I say, but realise there is something hidden under a wilted cress leaf.

I try to scoop it out with my index finger but give up as the dismembered head disappears into the cream cheese.

A waiter breezes over, stoops down and offers up a plate of untouched spring rolls with a giant plastic stag beetle glistening at the centre. He promises they don't have real beetles in them, but the trust is gone. Scout and Noah just look up at him like he's Skeletor.

'Let me see if there's some food in the foyer,' I say.

I feel my face flushing and instinctively look at Dyl to keep an eye on Scout. I hadn't packed any snacks because I'd assumed they wouldn't be serving up arthropods.

Walking through the selfie-taking throng, I nearly trip over @JabbaTheMutt lumbering through the crowd on a lead. He's a morbidly obese English Bulldog that has 515,000 followers. He doesn't know he's being followed by anyone other than his owner, a rake-thin man with pink hair and a deep mahogany tan that could be from Marbella or Boots. I wonder if the dog gets its own seat.

In the toilet queue is @Mother_minded. She's surrounded by bodies and looks like she wants to leave but that she needs a wee too desperately. I wonder if she's bothered about what they're saying on Influenza; if it's white noise to her or if she checks it obsessively and feels every insult like a slap.

I walk faster. Noah and Scout are hungry and the curtain's about to come up. I wonder if there's a corner shop nearby where I can get a couple of cereal bars. Something to make them squeal with excitement. There's a man dressed as a praying mantis, waving programmes around at the bottom of the stairs. He looks like he's having the time of his life, but takes a moment to direct me towards a staircase leading to the basement level and I start running as I hear the 'two minutes' warning.

There's a girl of about eighteen dressed in a white shirt and black tie alone at the basement bar next to the coat check. I buy a tub of honey-roasted nuts for £4.95 and four bottles of water for two quid each and thunder up the stairs. The crowds are thinning as I run back, and the lights are dimming as I see Dyl in the aisle, squatting down and talking to the kids. She sees me and there's a flicker of a smile as she stands up to relieve me of two of the damp bottles.

'They ate the spring rolls,' she says. 'I had to pull them apart to show them there wasn't a dead beetle inside, but then they scoffed the lot and the waiter gave them the toy from the middle.'

Noah proudly holds up the stag beetle as Scout looks on in awe, stroking its back like it's a rare Persian cat.

'We're going to share it,' says Scout. 'One week he'll be at my house and one week at Noah's.'

'But at Christmas, I have him, and at Easter, Scout does. So it's fair.'

They are at an age where justice is at the centre of everything.

'That's great,' I say, relieved, because I've taken Dyl to an event that has worms in the food and VIP dogs.

Scout is beaming in Noah's company, maybe the happiest I've seen her without sweets, toys or me.

We edge into our seats as a woman sitting in front of us scrolls through that familiar magenta Influenza screen.

'Can you please turn off your phones,' says a robotic voice across the tannoy.

The whole room lights up like a star constellation as people tap and then we're plunged into darkness. My shoulders relax into the musty velvet seat and I realise I'm three rows back from the dog.

The lights go up and we all blink and look at each other. I ask the kids what they thought.

'I didn't like the fire ant,' says Noah

'I didn't like the moth,' says Scout.

They both sound like they're discussing world news, not a musical about creepy-crawlies.

'What did you like?'

'THE BUTTERFLY,' they say in unison.

I have to agree it was a spectacle and worth the maggot starter. The whole stage was filled with colourful, floating silk, with a woman at the centre creating gentle waves. There was a trapeze and towers of bodies, and at least three times I thought someone might fall and die.

'It was beautiful,' says Dyl, and we walk silently together as the kids squabble over 'Macaroni', their beetle shell. They called him Macaroni in the way that kids just pair up two things they like.

We make our way out, edging behind a woman who looks like she's dressed up for Ladies Day at Ascot. She's got an air of authority and I think she's the mother of an influencer. I feel a tap on my shoulder.

'Sorry, are you Lo? From The Lo Down?'

She doesn't let me respond before saying, 'I LOVE your page.'

We're all suddenly blocking the entrance to the corridor and there's a crushed tempura cricket on the floor by Noah's foot.

'Hi!' I say, realising I don't know her. She continues to stand with us.

'What did you think?' she says, looking from Dyl to me.

'Loved it. This is my friend Dyl, by the way,' I say, hoping this woman will give me her name in return.

As I say the words, I wonder if I've spoken out of turn.

'Yeah, it was great,' Dyl says as she holds Noah's hand.

Scout slips her hand into mine too, like it's her own bespoke glove.

'What's your account?' the woman asks, eyes darting towards Dyl.

'I don't have one,' says Dyl.

'I sometimes wish I didn't have one,' she laughs, clasping two goody bags like they're gold bullion.

I look towards the exit and politely say goodbye as she makes a beeline for the fatigued PR. Our little convoy heads to the main foyer where the shivering lady in an African-print dress gives me a bag rammed with bug paraphernalia.

The cold October air fills our lungs as Scout and Noah run ahead and into a small doorway next to the theatre. It's already getting dark, and the West End is beginning to glow with light from shop windows and street lamps. Noah gallops Macaroni across the red-brick wall as Scout huffs, 'No, not like that,' like there's a right way for a plastic beetle to gallop.

Dyl and I walk in silence for a minute, the kids darting ahead to find walls to run the toy along.

'That was amazing,' says Dyl. 'Thanks so much for inviting us.'

'Sorry about the food. Just relieved they didn't serve butter-fly macaroons afterwards. Imagine the psychological damage.'

'No, they loved it in the end.'

Dyl opens her mouth to say more but is interrupted by Scout

letting out a loud cry. Noah is looking sheepishly on. She's tripped, and the tears are flowing as she holds her knee. We rush over, dumping our bags on the floor next to her.

'Do I have to go to hospital?' she whimpers, as tears drip onto her yellow rain mac and the chewing gum-smeared pavement.

'No, it's just a little scratch.'

I stoop down to her level to rub her knee better through her muddied jeans.

'Can I have a plaster?'

Her lower lip wobbles and she stares up at me with watery brown eyes.

'When we get home, nugget.'

'Squeeze me until the tears are all out, OK?'

I do, and pretend to drink the rest of her tears on her face until she's giggling like a loon, both of us forgetting for a moment that Dyl and Noah are there.

'I have a plaster,' Dyl says to Scout and she hands it to me.

I roll up her trouser leg and put it over the tiny graze, as Scout and Noah watch like I'm a master surgeon. Then they're fine again, and we move on along the street, the kids hand in hand as we feel the first drops of rain.

Then the drops get fatter and people scurry for cover as a tropical storm batters down.

The four of us stand and look at each other for a moment, not knowing where to go, and then run for the shelter of an awning outside a pub. The pavements turn slick with water and shimmer with the reflected glow of red brake lights from the London traffic.

'I'm soaking!' shouts Scout, eyes bright and laughing.

'Me too!' says Noah.

'We all are,' I tell them, wanting to soak up their energy. 'Let's wait here until it passes.'

We huddle beneath this temporary shelter and watch fat drops rattle off cars and splatter off tarmac. Dyl is drenched, the rain all soaked through her coat, and she shakes off water like a wet dog, igniting laughter in Noah and Scout. I never imagined what the women at the school gates would be like, but if this is my 'squad', it's going to be OK. Dyl has that rare combination of being interested in what you say but equally interesting. And she has suffered so much.

'I was thinking,' I say, 'that I could maybe help you.'

'What do you mean?'

'Help people to find your words. If we just set you up an Instagram for your blog. You don't have to do much. Just post snippets of your blog. I could link to you, and send some traffic over.'

She goes shy, quiet.

'I do have one, I just don't use it.'

'You do?'

'It just felt a bit daft, compared to yours. A bit silly. No one follows it.'

'But I can fix that.'

I can help her, and I should. Help pull her up. Support another woman to make her way through all the bollocks. I've been holding my phone in my coat pocket. I bring it out and open the app: 127 likes, thirteen comments, and thirty-eight new followers since we went into the theatre. I swipe to Influenza to check my thread is still dormant and realise I've stopped talking. She's just looking at me.

'What's your account?'

'It's @one__day__soon.'

I tap it in, and there it is: an anonymous account with twenty-three followers. A sunflower for the profile image, and a short bio:

Dylan Rayne. She/her.
Single working mother.
Read my work at onedaysoon.co.uk.

There is one post with an image of a supermarket shelf and a long caption.

> *I'm standing at the conveyor belt, rooted to the spot, the till glaring at me, my card declined. I'm not sure what this moment is making me feel. I'm not poor, I'm not a loser, I'm not shameless, I just have less than the person in front of me and the person behind me. One day soon they also might have less and then they won't be tutting or huffing or muttering as the cashier takes a packet of frozen peas off what I owe. And I'm one of the lucky ones. I have a roof and heat. There's no shame in struggling; there's shame in ignoring. Then you become part of the problem. Don't be one of the women who watch on.*
>
> *#endpoverty*

I feel like I shouldn't be reading it in front of her, but now she's watching to see what I say.

'Dyl, this is great. Your stuff is so great. I love that last line.'

She nods solemnly, her eyes looking up. Her cheeks are slightly flushed and her eyes flicker back to the ground.

'Everything you write makes me want to cry,' I tell her. 'It's like a slap in the face. These are things that are not being said.'

She wants this to work. She wants it to go further, and I can help her. After all she has suffered, losing her two men, I can help.

'Let me tag you. You might get a few hundred followers. More people will see your words.'

I screenshot her account and add text to a post.

Please read this brave new writer. No one writes about the daily reality of single motherhood like she does @one__day__soon.

I show her, to make sure she's happy.

'Can I?'

'OK.'

I send and she smiles, her shoulders dropping slightly as the rain eases back down to a trickle. I upload and we look at each other.

'We should get going,' she says. 'While the rain's stopped.'

I want to see if it's worked and she should too, but she's gone shy. She was so feisty when I first met her, but it's falling away so fast.

'Come on, Noah, let's go to the Tube.'

We gather the kids and walk up to Oxford Street, past a discount store filled with Halloween displays of evil pumpkins and demon masks and zombies dripping with blood.

'Noah, look,' says Scout, and we all have to stop.

'They're a bit scary,' he says.

The kids watch for a moment, transfixed by the ghouls staring out through their square little windows, and I turn to Lo.

'Do you want to check how it's going?'

'It's OK, I'll do it later.'

She's afraid, I think. She was so hard before, carrying around this big angry shell, but there's hurt inside – losing her dad, losing her partner. It would make anyone like that. And maybe now she's just a little scared about what people might think of her.

'It doesn't take long, usually,' I say.

She takes out her phone, flicks to Instagram. Her thumb glides down, and little rows of red appear.

Likes, follows, little taps of love.

'Oh wow,' she says, as her phone lights up.

18

DYLAN

It's half-term and Noah is watching telly. ChatTeam is ready to dial, but I can't look away from my phone, because every time I spin Instagram, there are more hearts and comments. It is glowing. I got nearly 900 followers the day Lo posted, 500 the next, and they've kept coming for two weeks. People keep tagging me to their mates and it just keeps growing. There are 3,274 now and every time I touch my phone there are more.

@Wanna-dem-too
Exactly! They're my kids! Why do I have to pay forty quid for their pictures!
@one__day__soon
Right!?!
@SweetC&roleRhymes
Pommes de terre de toms is sooooo tasty, thanks for the recipie!
@one__day__soon
Thanks! We love it. Can keep you going all day if you need to.

People are clicking through to the blog and reading my old stories and then coming back to tell me how much they love them. I didn't think there were that many women like me. They are listening and liking and I don't know how Lo keeps up. I never knew how much power she had sitting there in her pocket every day.

@KidKicksCancer!
I too was orphaned by suicide.

Oh. I wasn't exactly orphaned, it was just Dad, so . . .

@Kelly-anne-super-fan
Hey @Clairebear][1765, look at this one, she's got the photo rage too!

Maybe I'll answer her first.

'Mum, I'm hungry,' says Noah.

He's staring at PAW Patrol, practically horizontal, one hand in his tracksuit bottoms, the other picking his nose like a tiny teenager.

'Don't pick your nose please, Noah.'

He moves his finger away a few millimetres, but leaves it ready to rummage.

'Noah . . .'

He drops it to his chest.

Half-term is hard, because he gets a break, but I don't. He's barely been in school two months, but I've already got used to those hours when he's away. It's time for me to think, and make my calls. It's nearly six hours each day of being an independent grown-up. I miss him, and I think about him, but he's happy there and I can breathe, because for the first time since he was born, someone else is responsible too.

He talks about playing with other kids and how Ms Carole claps when they all have to listen and how the letter C is actually a 'curly kuh' and K is a 'kicking kuh' – like they're living things that he gets excited about – and I buzz inside when he talks about it.

But, also, it means I can work so much more. I generated twenty-seven follow-up calls last week and I've never done that many.

'Mummy, can I have a snack?'

'All right, Noh. You can have half an apple and maybe we'll go to the park later.'

'OK.'

His voice is dull. He's watched two hours of telly today and it's not even 10.00 a.m.

I take the last apple from the bowl by the sink and chop it in half, then chop each half into slices. The little paring knife is about the fanciest piece of kitchen kit in the flat. Everything else is blunt and battered old IKEA, but this is sharp and glides through like I'm on *MasterChef*. I reckon an old tenant left it by mistake. I put Noah's half in a bowl, walk over and lay the bowl on his belly, ruffle his hair.

'Thanks.'

I kiss two fingers and press them to his forehead, then go back to my laptop. Before I click ChatTeam, I send two emails.

Dear Sir or Madam,

For your consideration: a novel, *The Women Who Watch On*. And for examples of my published works, please visit onedaysoon.co.uk or on Instagram @one__day__soon.

Yours truly,
Dylan Rayne

I've been adding @one__day__soon since Lo tagged me. I want them to see that people like what I have to say.

I go back to my inbox and there's one new work email, sent to All Team from my line manager. It's all the usual pep.

> Take full advantage of core calling hours . . . welcome to new affiliates . . . hydration becomes more important as Christmas approaches . . . And congratulations to Dylan Rayne of London and South East, who generated twenty-seven follow-up calls in a single week, a new personal record for her! You are on fire, Dylan, keep up the great work!

Jeez, Dyl, the whole bloody world loves you. I flick to the blog, and check my latest draft post, scheduled to go live tonight.

I'll put it up at 20:30 – then post on Instagram so people know. Everyone looks at their phone the minute the kids are down and Lo says midweek is best for engagement.

And the thing I've found is that the sadder my stories, the more people like them.

One Day Soon
20:30, 16 October

Moving by Bus

I left because he locked me in the bathroom.

I drank sink water and ate toothpaste and was thirty-eight weeks pregnant and he left me there for two days.

We had a smaller flat this time, and he was calmer because I had no friends by then.

And because I had his baby in me.

'Definitely just one in there, is it?'

164

He didn't want a baby, but he didn't want condoms either and sometimes the pill isn't enough.

But it made him softer for a bit. He made me soup some days.

Then, one morning, I found out about the loans.

Twelve grand on credit cards, a bank loan, a payday lender, my name on everything.

So I shouted at him and I cried and he said calm down, think of the baby, but I kept shouting like I'd never done before.

And when I went to the toilet, he locked me in. Took the key from the kitchen drawer and turned it in the old metal latch.

I was there with my knickers round my ankles and I was fat and slow. I rattled the door and called his name until the front door slammed.

And for a minute, I thought, he's left me here to die in this little room with no window and a rattling fart fan in the ceiling full of dust and germs and making me sick.

He hates me so much, he has left me here to die.

He hates my voice and my shape and the life inside me, so he will walk away and let me starve.

I pulled at the door and I pushed it and I rattled it and I screamed.

And after a while my voice was worn and I had no more tears left so I made a little bed: one towel for a pillow, one for a blanket.

I could smell the dampness on my shoulder and it made me shiver.

I rested my belly on my arm and when I couldn't feel my arm anymore, I turned over. I did that all night, my ribs and elbows pressed on the lino floor, and cried all the next morning until my eyes ran dry again and my cheeks were like crusts. When it felt like night again, I remade my bed.

He came back the next day.

'Oh my God, I'm so sorry, I didn't know you were in there.'

He made me soup and put me in our bed and said I should have called out.

'You've got to think of the little one, Dilly.'

He wrapped me in blankets and I had the curtains closed all day and didn't speak. When I went to the toilet, I held the door open, but I couldn't reach it from the bath, so I didn't wash.

We were like that for a week, and then he got bored and went drinking.

'Right moper, you are.'

And that afternoon I felt my body clench and knew I had to go.

An ambulance would take me local and he would find me there, so I walked out and got the bus as far as I could.

My waters broke on the North Circular and I made a funny noise, but the bus was packed and there's always someone making funny noises on buses.

When I got off, the seat was wet.

It made me feel bad for whoever sat there next.

When we get on buses now, I always make sure my boy checks the seat before he sits down.

19

NOVEMBER

LO

London cabs always make me feel important. Staring out of the window as the capital whips by is like having a private viewing of your favourite city.

It's a bright Friday morning and we cut through the leafy grandeur of Barnsbury, through the post-industrial polish of Somers Town, and the driver drops me at a place called Canal Studios. The name is styled in an art-deco wrought-iron font against a white wall. If I squint, it could be a bit of Hollywood glamour, rather than an old industrial estate round the back of King's Cross.

At reception is a woman with a clipboard, dressed in tight blue jeans and a plain black tee. She is willowy and slight and can't be over twenty. I instantly feel out of place, like a *hausfrau* that's stepped into Chinawhite. My lungs tighten and I clench my jaw, waiting for the girl to look up from her phone.

'Are you Lois Knox?'

'Yes. Well, just Lo. Short for Lois. Like Lois Lane.'

This is my stock reply. It's meant to break the ice, but her smile flashes and collapses as she begins to walk ahead.

'Great. Just follow me.'

She stalks through some strip-lit corridors as I trot behind, turning my phone over in my coat pocket. This is the day, and I can feel little rushes surge up from my belly, part anxiety, part thrill. I imagine old colleagues at Darby Cooper seeing me on a panty-liner advert and smile.

We turn a corner and the girl with the clipboard pushes open double doors to reveal a vast white space. There must be a dozen people clanking around with kit or deep in conversation. In one corner is a green sofa and armchairs, and settled there with coffees are a few other women, each illuminated by the glow of their phones.

This is where I'll make my national television debut.

'You'll just need make-up first,' says the girl.

She leads me to an alcove that has a vast mirror with lights all around it and a make-up table and chair.

'This is Niamh, she'll take care of you.'

Niamh nods and I sit down. She has a case of make-up that looks like a miniature stadium, and is considering my face like a mechanic with a misfiring engine.

'They said I could just do my usual make-up,' I tell her.

'Yes,' she says. 'It's fine. We'll just go over the top.'

She smells of aniseed and talcum powder. To my left, someone is steaming a rail of clothes.

I couldn't sleep last night. My mind just kept firing, and I don't think I got more than four hours. With the glare of lights around the mirror, I can see how tired I look. My eyes are a little more sunken, like they're rolling back into my skull to get a little rest.

'Everyone's having a red lip,' says Niamh, 'but what are you thinking about the eyes. Maybe something smoky?'

She sways from foot to foot, weighing up the possibilities with the soiled canvas in front of her.

I sink back into the squeaky chair, my phone hot on my thigh, and say, 'Sure, sounds great.'

I flick to Influenza as she changes my face. A new comment is on my thread and my heart clenches slightly as Niamh sweeps foundation under my eyes.

CarlaCowabunga says: She's starting to grate a bit. Lots of virtue-signalling but very little action. Like what is she actually doing other than posing with her tits out?

I swipe away as Niamh trails a fine layer of glue across my eyelids and gently pats a fake eyelash onto each one. The corner of my left eye is briefly glued shut and she uses a comb to separate the lashes until I can blink and see again.

'OK?'

I nod and Niamh smiles. She pulls out the blusher and I close my eyes once more to let her work. She dusts and dabs and it's a relief to be in darkness. My palms are sweaty and my mouth dry. I can feel my lips cracking under the lipstick.

When I left this morning, I gave Scout a hug and told her to have a great day, then I gave Johno a peck, but it was like kissing a colleague. He went for my cheek, not my lips, like a schoolboy kissing his nan.

I can feel Niamh working my brows with a brush, and the soft movement helps me drift for a while.

'There we go.'

I open my eyes and she's gone heavy. I look like I'm about to hit the West End stage.

'We need lots of definition for the lights.'

'Yes, great, thanks.'

'Now, Elliott will be with you for hair.'

Niamh steps away and Elliott steps in.

'Hello there,' he says, smiling at me via the mirror.

Elliott begins cupping the ends of my hair, bouncing it just above my shoulders and fanning it out with his fingers. I know it is thin. I know when he pulls his fingers away, curly brown strands will float away from the root.

'You've got a lovely colour.'

'I had it dyed recently. Some sneaky greys were coming through.'

Elliott is kind enough to look surprised.

'That's very early.'

And I suppose it is.

'So what shall we do? Maybe just a bit of volumising?'

He's running parted fingers across my scalp and it's the closest I've come to a massage in months.

'I'm in your hands,' I tell him.

He begins to tease my hair up with his fingers and gently lets it fall.

'We'll just add a little volume,' he says.

Elliott pulls out a curling iron and I pull out my phone. He very gently works my hair around the large barrel, holding it for a few seconds and then letting it tumble.

I scroll as he works around my head, and I have a new DM from someone called @iamlina1991.

'I don't know if you will even see this, but I have no one to turn to. I have lost eight babies and I want to thank you for your openness. My family don't see it as loss, they see it as failure. I don't know why I'm here because you are a stranger, but I am praying for our rainbow babies and when you said 'I lost a small part of myself' it resonated so much. Because I feel like I'm losing myself. Please don't share this with anyone. His name was Oscar. He was born sleeping yesterday at twenty-two weeks. Lina x'

And there is a picture of her boy, Oscar, with his eyes firmly shut.

Eyelids so thin, like wet paper.

Eyelids so thin it feels like the eyes are peering right through to look at me.

Like they can see through that baking-paper skin, even though they will never see anything.

And he is wrapped in white cotton, all folded to a little V below his tiny chin.

And he is so still.

So still and perfect, but his skin so pale.

The faintest sky blue, but for thin dark lips, like a person unfinished.

I close my eyes, but Oscar is still there, the image of his closed mouth burned onto the back of my eyelids.

'Oh my God, how cute,' says Elliott.

I look back at him in the mirror and he's releasing a curl of my hair.

'Bit too new for me, though. I just think they're scary that little.'

He wraps another strand around the curler.

'This is terrible, but I've got a mate who says he won't even pick them up under a month because they still smell of vagina!'

My stomach knots and I look back at the picture of little Oscar.

My arms feel light and empty and my fingers go loose around the phone and I twitch to grasp it so it can't slip from my hand because I don't want him to fall on the floor.

And then I wonder if my baby had eyelashes. If he or she was more than 'foetal matter', and my heart and womb ache.

'Nearly done. I'm just going to brush it through to give some natural bounce.'

Elliott reaches for a paddle brush and pulls it through my hair and at the end of every sweep, a few wispy hairs trail behind.

I look back at Oscar and I wonder how his skin feels.

I wonder how long she could keep him warm.

'Are we all done?'

It's the girl with the clipboard.

'Yes, she's all done.'

Elliott smiles and steps away, and the girl with the clipboard points to the sofas, where a cluster of paper coffee cups is growing around a platter of dry melon slices.

'You can wait over here,' she says

'What's your name?'

'Carly!' She smiles like she's not used to being asked and I see a tiny brace on her top front teeth. I want to hold on to her, just for a moment, but she's done with me, too. 'If you just have a seat, wardrobe will need you in a minute.'

I sit down and I can feel Oscar's weight in my arms.

There are eight of us around the table, and we must be the ones going in front of the camera, because we all have inch-thick make-up on. We are all different colours and shapes and ages and I recognise a few faces from Instagram, but there is no one I know. I might be the oldest. I guess panty-liner demographics have a natural cut-off.

I hold up my phone, but I can't look again. I just smile at everyone around the table.

Today I am selling sustainable panty liners, and they have asked me to be myself, even though I don't know who that is. I remember her at dinner parties, telling stories that would lift the room. I would see eyes flashing, jaws aching, chairs creaking as people leaned back with laughter. I remember her smile as she told boys what she wanted from them. Outside pubs, inside clubs, on top of hostel beds. I remember her making

172

cards for friends, wiping tears from drunk strangers in toilets, never forgetting a birthday and going to bed with make-up on.

So I can fake it, put on a smile, say what they want me to say.

Today could change my life. I will earn money promoting something that helps women.

I can make our little family more secure and be there at the school gates, and Scout will see that happen. She will know I made it happen. She will know that success isn't in the hands of men in boardrooms wondering why there are so few women sitting beside them.

But I also can't leave Lina, because there was a moment when she let little Oscar go.

There was a moment when she held him in her arms and he turned cold, and a moment when they took him away.

And I don't know if they had to force her.

Or how they got him out of her arms.

If anyone was there with her or if she was alone.

I don't know if the nurses were kind or impatient or how long they give you.

'The Lo Down?'

A woman stands before me in bright orange dungarees.

'Yes?'

'Hey! Let's get you dressed.'

She opens her arms wide, fingers splayed.

I stand and walk to her and she walks quickly towards the rails of clothes.

'They've asked for colour blocking but no reds. How do you feel about emerald?'

'I feel fine.'

She flicks through the rack and pulls out three pieces: a purple jumpsuit, a green maxi dress and a puffball piece.

She looks at me and sets the puffball aside.

'You have such wonderful shape, we don't need to add to it. I'm a rectangle, so I need structuring, but either of these two should just tumble off your form.'

She pulls back the curtains on a temporary changing room and hands me the two outfits as I head in. She swishes the curtain back and I feel my stomach roll. I think I might be sick and I step over to a wastepaper bin in the corner. I can feel sweat beading on my forehead and I need to sit, but there's no stool so I sit on the floor.

I breathe slowly three times.

I'm worried that if I stand I might fall, and I breathe three times more.

'Are you OK, honey?'

I can see the stylist's white trainers just outside.

'Yes. Great. These are lovely.'

She steps away and I push myself upwards to stand. In the mirror, I can see the sweat pimpling on top of the concealer. I don't have a tissue, so I press very gently with the tips of my fingers, then wipe them on the curtain, where they leave a faint stain. I put on the maxi dress and step out.

'Oh! That really suits you. Now, let's try the jumpsuit.'

'I really like this.'

'Are you sure?'

'This is great.'

'Well, OK, then!'

She smiles and steps aside, waving me back towards the sofas.

'You've been the easiest yet!'

I want to step outside and feel the coolness of the air. I want to take the time to reply to a woman who birthed and lost a baby in a few minutes yesterday afternoon.

'Hi! I'm Luna.'

There's a woman in front of me who is at least six foot and has added three inches with thick-soled black boots. She has a perfectly straight black bob and a star tattooed on one earlobe. But she's wearing a thin white dress that looks like she should be in the cast of *A Midsummer Night's Dream*.

'Hi, I'm Lo.'

I smile and hold out my hand, which she shakes.

'You ready to shine for period poverty?'

She smiles as she says this – a huge, clownish grin of excitement.

'Definitely,' I smile back.

And then I just stop, because I have nothing to say.

'I'm on after you,' says Luna.

'Cool!'

On the set, a props man is on a ladder straightening up a neon sign that says, 'Blood on Your Hands'.

One of my false eyelashes is coming loose and I turn away from Luna to pat it back into place. She doesn't say anything else, so we stand in silence as the other women begin to gather around us.

The props man is lining up eight pots of red paint beneath the sign.

I feel a weight press down on my shoulder and it's a young guy with a roller, taking fluff off my dress, like I'm a dog about to be shown at Crufts.

A woman in a short red dress and red trainers strides towards us all.

'Hi guys, I'm Imani, the creative director.'

A few women say, 'Hi, Imani,' and she smiles. It's a magnanimous smile, like she's used to people singing out her name.

'So, you all know why you're here,' she says as the group blankly nods. 'Today we are doing something bold and dynamic.

You have each been chosen for your unique, digital voice and we are so excited to have you on board for this campaign. Excuse the pun, but you all look bloody wonderful.'

She continues smiling and I wonder how many times they've used that. She introduces Emma, the marketing director at WeAreFemForm, the woman paying everyone's wages.

'I just want to thank you for being a part of the FF journey,' she says. 'We're so excited to have you here, helping us to make change on such a fundamental issue.'

Everyone smiles.

A man steps forward, clapping his hands once, loudly.

'So, I guess it's me next.'

He's wearing a red baseball cap, jeans and a thin jacket that zips up to his chin.

'I'm Ayan, I'm the director today. We're really excited to have you all here. I know you're used to directing yourselves, so we're going to have a very free shoot.'

He pauses, allows us to appreciate his magnanimity.

'We'll really give you the chance to express yourselves and share what you're feeling. We're going to start with the solo clips, then have some raw moments at the end with everybody together. That's when it might get a bit messy.'

He smiles and turns to look at the paint pots.

'Now, just relax, and we'll get started in a minute.'

He smiles and walks away; a sign for the crowd to slowly disperse.

Imani puts her hand on my shoulder and I jerk back.

'Sorry! Didn't mean to scare you.'

'No, that's OK. I was just getting ready.'

'Well, we're really glad to have you. I love what you're doing. I pushed you to the client personally.'

'Oh, thanks.'

'How did you find the experiment? It's a bit much, I know, but it felt so important.'

'The experiment?'

'The period-poverty experiment.'

She looks confused, and perhaps I do, too.

'Where you spend a full cycle without sanitary products?' she says.

I'm expecting her to laugh, but she looks at me very seriously.

'Um, no. I didn't . . . No one told me.'

'Didn't you get the briefing?'

'I got an overview: it's WeAreFemForm, it's period poverty, there's a car booked for 8.00 a.m.'

'Oh. OK. Well the idea was that you go for one cycle without sanitary products, to experience period poverty, and now you tell us all about it.'

'Oh. But I haven't.'

'Yes. I'm not sure it will work without that.'

'Oh.'

'Maybe you could just improvise a bit?'

'Just pretend?'

'I really pushed to get you on this. It would be a real help. And we have lots more projects coming.'

Carly appears next to us.

'Hi, Lo, we've got you first.'

There's a soundman next to her with headphones and a mic, which he hands to me and I thread up inside my dress and pull out of the top. He delicately clips the mic to the dress near my breast, fingers out like a conductor so he doesn't touch anything he shouldn't. He hands me the mic pack and it hoists my dress up from ankle height to knee height.

'Just put this on the floor while you're talking.'

'You'll be great,' says Imani. 'Just be yourself.'

Carly leads me onto the stage as I clutch the mic pack and the lights beam down. There's one camera pointed directly at me, another to my side. The set is bright white and powerfully lit as the lights around us dim and everyone falls silent. I set the mic pack on the floor between my feet. Ayan is staring at a monitor and steps forward to clap his hands once.

'Hi. It's Lo, right?'

'Yes.'

'Great. Could you just give us a big shake?'

'A shake?'

'Yeah, roll your shoulders, shake your arms, get that stiffness out.'

So I do. I give a little shake and smile like I'm performing in a school play.

Ayan turns to talk over his shoulder.

'Niamh, could we get a little . . .'

Niamh appears and dusts my forehead with more foundation to cover the forming sheen as Ayan walks back to his monitor by the main camera.

Then she presses my eyelash more firmly onto my upper lid. I think about Oscar's eyelids, born shut, never to open. Lina will know I've seen her message. She might be alone. She might be waiting for me to reply.

'So, Lo.'

Ayan claps again.

'Carly's going to be standing just next to this camera, and she will ask you some questions. Just reply straight to her, like you're talking to a friend.'

I look towards her, but she's in the dark and I'm lit up and I can barely see her face. Someone calls for quiet, and it's just me and her and a dozen people staring in silence.

'Lo. Tell me how you feel about period poverty.'

'How I feel?'

'How does period poverty make you feel? How do you feel about the fact that forty-nine per cent of young girls have missed an entire day of school because of their period?'

'Bad.'

They all stand and wait for something more.

'Period poverty is terrible.'

Ayan leans around the monitor

'You can let it all out here, Lo. We've got loads of time. Just let it flow and we'll cut it later. Just be your authentic self.'

There's silence again. My body feels clammy, but my face feels so warm.

'Period poverty is a shame . . .'

They wait, but nothing comes. I feel like I've been standing here for twenty minutes, and in the shadows all I can see are the tiny blue veins across Oscar's eyelids.

'Period poverty is a shame no woman should have to endure. Period poverty is a shame for a nation, but not its women. Period poverty is something that a country inflicts on its women, not something women inflict on themselves. What choice is it if a woman must choose between feeding herself and managing her menstrual cycle? No woman should—'

'Sorry, sorry.'

It's Ayan.

'Niamh, could we just . . .'

Niamh appears and dusts the sweat on my brow. She stands back and looks and then she does it again.

'Thanks, Niamh. That was really strong, Lo. Really great. Just remember we're not political: we don't give blame, but we do empathise. Carly . . .'

'So, Lo. How did your experience with period poverty make you feel?'

'Sorry,' says Imani, a voice attached to a face I can't quite see, 'maybe we could focus on how you feel for those living with period poverty? You're such an empathetic voice, Lo. Just be your natural self.'

'Sure.'

I clear my throat. Relax my shoulders.

'Although we need this first-person,' says Ayan. 'How it feels for *you*.'

'Anything else?'

I try to smile

'No. When you're ready . . .'

'How does period poverty make me feel? It makes me feel sad. It makes me feel like we're letting all those women down. It makes me feel that when a woman misses work, or school, or an interview because she's so embarrassed that she can't afford sanitary products, she is penalised for being a woman. And when that happens to one woman, it happens to us all. There's no shame in struggling. There's no shame in bleeding. There's shame in ignoring. Then you become part of the problem. Don't be one of the women who watch on.'

There's a silence.

'Do you want more?'

'No, that's great. Really lovely,' says Ayan. 'We just need the tagline now.'

'Hi, Lo,' says Carly. 'If you could just say straight to camera: I've experienced period poverty. Let's end it today.'

I do exactly as she asks.

20

DYLAN

It is cold but bright in the playground, a pretty Friday at the end of Noah's first week back, and these days feel like they clean the air. Every breath flows in from my nose to my lungs to my fingertips and as I wait for his class, I flick to my phone. Spin, watch, wait . . . eighteen new followers and a little flutter in my belly. That's 5,912.

I tap the profile pics one by one and peek into their lives. There are so many like mine. They're not in houses, they're in flats. No Cath Kidston and Le Creuset, just Tesco and chipped mugs.

There's a new direct message from @hopingwaiting247.

'When I see what you write, I know I can cope.'

'Moving by Bus' has gone crazy. The views counter on the blog has hit 20,000, and all these messages came through. Women like me. Women who had to run, or who want to. All telling me how much I helped make them feel stronger, made them feel brave.

This is what words should do. Lift us up, help us. Lo got me started, but now a new audience is finding me. She has an army of thousands just carried around in her pocket and they're telling their friends, who are telling theirs, and they all like what I'm writing.

It is new and exciting and mine.

Noah spots me and is released, running over the rainbow mural on the playground floor as I squat down. He clamps himself around my neck, nearly knocking me over.

'What's for tea?'

'Tomato soup.'

I can already see the orange moustache on his upper lip as he does his impression of an old man.

'Can I have hairy cheese on it?'

'Only if you eat a whole clementine after. Today we're having orange and yellow food.'

'OK. Can I make the cheese like a face on the top of the soup?'

'Yes.'

I bought a chunky bloomer this morning, which has made me more excited than it should. I will grill big chunks, because that way it soaks up more soup. It's tragic, but this is what moves me. In a moment of loopy excitement earlier this week, I bought some activated charcoal biscuits for three quid. I tried one and it tasted like pebbles. It made me wonder if there's some global wellness guru saying, 'Ha-ha, let's see if they'll eat rocks!' and, like mugs, we do. I spent a meal's budget on some biscuits I don't like, but it doesn't matter, because I am moving forward. I have 5,912 followers and I'm helping people cope. I haven't sold any water coolers this week, but my pipeline is good.

We head towards the red metal gates and my phone rings in my pocket. It's a jolt. Who phones?

The name flashes up: Lo.

'Hello?'

'Hi, Dyl.'

'Hi, you all right?'

She sounds like she's running underwater and then the line cuts out. The number comes through again.

'Sorry, the connection is rubbish. I'm really sorry, but would you mind waiting with Scout? I'm coming from this shoot, but there's traffic and she gets upset if she's the last one—'

And then she's gone again.

'Who was that?'

'Scout's mummy.'

'Are we going to play?'

He looks up like a dog wanting a treat.

'You can't have playdates every day, Noh.'

'Awwwww.'

His voice sounds like a trumpet-player running out of steam. But why can't he have playdates every day? Maybe it's time for Scout to come to ours.

'We can wait with Scout, though, because her mummy's late.'

We turn around and walk back against the tide of parents. While we loiter, I try to play rock-paper-scissors with Noah, but he just wants to smile and wave at Scout. Eventually the tide of parents becomes a trickle, and there's just us, Scout and Ms Carole. She looks in my direction.

'Is everything OK?'

'Yes. Scout's mum is late and she asked me to wait.'

'Oh, I see. Your mummy will be here soon, Scout.'

She looks at Scout, who smiles up at her a little unconvinced.

'We do have a nominated persons list,' says Ms Carole.

'OK?'

'You can nominate another parent to collect your child if you're late.'

'Oh, I see.'

Then I hear a frantic clopping of heels over concrete. We look around and Lo is trotting across the playground. She arrives in a bounce of freshly done curls and this massive green dress. Her dark hair sits heavy across her shoulders, shining like something out of a conditioner ad.

'Hello! I'm so sorry!'

She smiles at everyone and Scout runs towards her for a big hug.

Her make-up is thick and her lashes make her look like she's about to go on stage.

'God, ignore my face,' she says, putting her hands up, and I realise I must have been staring. 'They cake it on when there's lights and then you forget and find yourself on the school run looking like a Kardashian.'

'It doesn't look that bad.'

'Dyl, I look like a clown. We can call it, and it's OK.'

She laughs a bit manically and turns to Ms Carole to say sorry again.

'It happens. We do ask parents to try to be sure they arrive on time. Staff often have lots to do after the school day is finished.'

The teacher is actually telling her off, like she's the kid.

'Yes, I'm sorry. I feel like it's always me!'

'As I was telling Noah's mum, some parents nominate other parents to collect their children in their absence.'

'Great! We could do that, couldn't we, Dyl?'

She looks at me. There's a false eyelash falling off.

'Just in case, I mean,' she says. 'So Ms Carole doesn't have to wait. And I'll do it for Noah?'

The teacher turns to me, smiles gently.

'They're such good pals these two, we can barely keep them apart in class.'

They're acting like it's the most natural thing in the world. Like it doesn't matter who collects him. But I will never be late for Noah.

'Maybe.'

Ms Carole smiles. Then she turns around and we're free to go.

'I'm so sorry,' Lo says. 'Terrible day.'

'That's OK.'

We start to walk towards the gates. We're the last parents and the caretaker is waiting to lock up. He looks at me and smiles, and ignores Lo completely.

'I really am so sorry to make you wait,' she says. 'I just keep being late and Scout's getting really hacked off with it.'

'It's fine, we had no plans.'

'Do you want to come by for tea?'

She says this like she's excited, and the kids start jumping up and down.

'Ummm . . .'

'I've got a lasagna.'

There is something desperate about her, something pleading.

'It doesn't have to be for long, if you don't fancy,' she says, the enthusiasm in her voice draining, like she's scared we'll slip away.

Noah grabs my hand and starts pulling on it, gazing up at me with wild hope.

'Only if you're sure.'

'I am SO sure.'

We get to Lo's and the kids sprint upstairs while we head to the kitchen.

'Here she is,' she says, pulling a giant lasagna from the fridge and talking about it like an old mate. 'Johno made it last night, but then I was busy and we never got round to eating.'

She slides it into the oven. There's a laundry basket on the floor and she darts for it like it might explode, sliding it to the double back doors.

Then she stands and looks at me hopefully.

'Do you fancy a drink?'

She's already walking over to the fridge and there's something frantic about her. Like there's an electric charge running through her.

'I mean, I know it's a bit early, but it's also Friday,' she says, smiling at me. 'And it's been a long day,' she adds, peeling off an eyelash.

'Yeah, it has.'

But my day's been fine. It has been good. I have had a normal-length day.

'White wine?' She holds up a half-full bottle like I'm choosing a paint swatch. 'Or gin?'

'Wine is great, thanks, Lo.'

The oven clock says 3.45 p.m., but she pours the wine heavily. Then she drops the fake eyelashes in the bin, wipes off excess red lipstick with a square of kitchen towel and looks more human as she sits down.

'How was your day?' she asks.

'Fine. I tried to sell water coolers to a disgruntled office manager in the West Midlands. How about you?'

'Erm, I sold myself.' She laughs. 'Just the soul today, not the tits and arse.'

I laugh back.

'And Insta's been amazing,' I tell her.

'Has it?'

'Yeah. Since you tagged me. It's gone mad, people love it, I've got nearly 6,000 followers.'

She looks stunned, like she can't compute it.

'Really? I hadn't even looked . . .'

'Yeah, loads of comments and likes and people reading the old blog posts. It's mad; thank you so much.'

'Wow. That's . . . Six thousand in barely three weeks is amazing. I don't think I ever got that.'

She smiles, but looks surprised. Like maybe she didn't realise how much she could help. Or how much I would grow.

'God,' she says, 'I wish I'd had a big account to tag me at the beginning.' And she smiles, like maybe it's not a dig and she's genuinely amazed, but it still sits there like a little reminder: she gave this to me.

'Honestly, Lo, you've helped so much. I've been doing this for years and no one's cared, but one tag from you and people love it. You've really helped.'

'Good, that's great. I mean, your stuff about your dad is amazing, so it should be seen.'

'Well, it's all down to you, so thanks.'

She's quiet for a moment, then raises her glass.

'Here's to One Day Soon.'

We clink glasses and each take a sip.

'What were you doing today that's got you looking all fancy?'

'It was a shoot for a sustainable sanitary towel. They're washable and reusable, and five per cent of their profit goes to charity. It was good on paper, but the reality was eight influencers dipping their hands in red paint in the name of period poverty.'

Her voice lowers again slightly when she says 'poverty'. She senses the awkwardness, her eyes flicker down.

She takes a bigger sip of wine, the smears on her glass

highlighted by the afternoon light, then goes to the freezer and starts rummaging around.

Noah and Scout are now playing a game upstairs that involves a loud thud every two minutes. Lo plonks ice in my glass without asking and turns to her phone.

Maybe she wants to check One Day Soon.

She taps and stares, swipes her thumb. I can't see what she's looking at, but it's taken her out of the room. She's somewhere else now, in other conversations, eyes vacant, finger and thumb twirling a strand of her hair. I reach for my phone to make it less awkward. Her face looks weighed down and her eyes narrow.

'You must get a lot of messages,' I say.

'Yeah, it's quite intense at times. I love hearing from people, but today there was a woman whose baby was stillborn. I don't know what to say to make her feel better. It's not just a "sorry hun".'

She looks shaken and I want to touch her, put a hand on her shoulder, but I don't know if I can. I pour her more wine and then some for me. I can feel my muscles loosen a bit and I wonder if she can, too.

'His name was Oscar.' She takes a gulp and looks at me. 'Imagine the loneliness of having no one but a stranger on the internet to say that to: "My baby died and no one else cares, but I thought you might." I can't stop thinking about her.'

There's a silence and it's my turn to fill it.

'That is heartbreaking.'

She doesn't respond, so I go again.

'That kind of loneliness must be terrible.'

I say it like it's unimaginable, but really, who would I tell if something terrible happened? Mrs Younis? I don't think she knows it, but it's probably Lo.

She just takes another sip of wine, so I do, too. It's so cold now, it glides down like there's no booze in it at all. We can hear running upstairs and it seems to shake her loose.

'God, sorry!'

She gives a short hard laugh and shakes her head, like she's trying to bring herself back to life. Then she jags forward, almost shouting:

'Anyway, that's amazing about One Day Soon.'

'Thanks. It's going OK.'

I smile, not wanting to do any more showing off.

We hear a thump, like a foot stamping upstairs, and Noah shouts, 'PLEASE' very loudly.

We exchange a look and both walk to the stairs. He is not a boy who shouts, so I just march up ahead of her, but then I slow halfway, because it feels invasive even though my own son is there. I've never been upstairs before, to where they wash and sleep, but I know exactly what their bedroom looks like from the pictures I've seen on Instagram, pictured them in it, wondered how they sleep.

Lo creaks up behind me, holding two beakers of juice for the kids. We get to Scout's room and they both look sheepish. They stand next to each other, faces staring down at the Lego-covered carpet.

'Scout won't let me feed her fish,' says Noah quietly.

'It's because I've already fed him,' says Scout, looking upset.

'But he can have a snack,' says Noah.

I squat down to his level.

'Noah, it's Scout's fish and it can't have too much food otherwise its tummy will get sore.'

He nods forlornly and looks towards Scout.

Lo holds out the beakers.

'Are you two thirsty?'

They nod and take the drinks and go back to pulling everything out of the grey wicker toy box and onto the floor.

'Noh, be careful with Scout's stuff,' I say. 'You'll have to tidy up everything you take out, OK?'

He nods and carries on digging for a toy he doesn't yet know he wants.

'It's OK,' says Lo. 'Whatever keeps them quiet.'

We head downstairs, the steps creaking as the smell of lasagna seeps out of the kitchen. She looks at me like we're spies.

'One more glass before we feed them?'

We settle Noah and Scout next to each other on the sofa to watch TV while lasagna settles in their bellies. Scout has two straws under her upper lip and turns to Noah like she's a walrus, and he laughs like it's the best thing he's ever seen.

We go back to the kitchen and Lo fills my glass without asking, pouring the rest of the second bottle into her own. We're drunk now, woozy, light and warm. But at the nice level. All feels well and I haven't felt like this in a long time.

The smell of the lasagna is making me hungry and I want to take a spoon to the burnt pasta in the corner of the dish. Lo reads my mind, hands me a fork without speaking, and we both dig at the remains straight from the baking tray.

The oven clock says it's 6.42 p.m., which is past bathtime, but the kids are happy and my shoulders have eased. For the first time in months, my mind just drifts and I try not to think about getting Noah home and into bed.

My whole body feels warm with alcohol and I realise Lo's been speaking in a whispered tone for a while, even though there is no one other than two distracted kids and a distant goldfish to hear us. It makes me lean in and I find my focus landing on a little piercing on the inside of her ear. It's so small I've never seen it before.

'We haven't had sex for two weeks,' she says.

'My vagina is hibernating,' I say.

She laughs. It's a big, honest laugh. A huge squeal that makes you want to hear it again.

'Honestly,' I say, 'if I saw a naked man right now, I wouldn't know what to do with him.'

And I wouldn't, I don't think. There's been no one since JD. Four years a lonely nun.

Lo titters a bit, like she's expecting me to continue, but I pull back. I don't want her to ask me about men. She gives me a second and then she starts again.

'I mean, I want to have sex. I like having sex, but my body is such a state. There's this pocket of skin hanging over my C-section scar that basically makes me feel like I have a fourth hole.'

I smile for her.

'Johno has probably shagged it,' she continues, 'thinking it's my fanny.'

'Well at least there's contact. All I've got is impure thoughts about the school caretaker.'

She does her big laugh again and it feels good. I am entertaining an adult with my words. And then she goes quiet, as she realises why that's all I've got. Poor widow Dyl with the dead partner.

I go to fill our glasses, but the bottle is empty.

'I can fix that,' she says.

'No, we've had two bottles! I should get Noah back.'

'What! They're fine. Just stay here tonight. He can top and tail with Scout and we've got a spare room for you. In fact, you and I can top and tail and Johno can have the spare room. It's Friday, so he'll be late and pissed.'

'No, it's OK. We're ten minutes away.'

She leans forward, looks at me very seriously, frowns and shakes her head.

'Let's have a look at how happy our children are.'

We get up and head towards the lounge. Lo has her finger to her pursed lip, even though I'm not making a sound. On the green velvet sofa, Scout and Noah are curled up like two kittens, with *SpongeBob SquarePants* now on the TV. We stand in the doorway in silence, just staring for a moment, and I flinch as her left arm slips inside my right, under my pit, and she wraps our forearms together, pulling me tight to her side like we're a little old couple.

'We cannot interrupt that scene,' she whispers.

No one ever holds me except Noah.

I look her in the eye and she grins.

Then she fetches another bottle and we return to smudged wine glasses in the kitchen.

It's past 8.00 p.m. and we're eating crisps and the last bits of a pizza, both sipping more slowly now. She has changed into jeans and a T-shirt and wiped off all the make-up, and you can see that she is pretty but that there's a goodness to her as well.

She feels like a nice person and I don't know how I ever got her so wrong. She is vulnerable and caring and she wants to help and I just want to hug her. We've been talking about Broxton ward again, and I don't want tonight to end yet.

'My scar looks like someone just opened a tin and forgot about it,' I tell her, 'but, luckily, there's enough bush to hide it.'

'I was so scared about my engorged vagina I nearly dialled 999,' says Lo. 'It was as big as a fist.'

As she holds her fist up, we both screech and my arms flop to my side as I look at her.

'I've been shaving mine all off recently because I couldn't be arsed with the faff of waxing anymore,' she says. 'But now it looks like a plucked turkey.'

She leans back, pulls the band of her jeans down and shows me her C-section scar, as casually as if it was a chipped nail.

'I don't think you'll even be able to see my scar through the growth.' I pull my jeggings down and show a jagged line just above a dark mass of hair. 'Look at this monster muff!'

She howls with laughter, rocks back in her chair and tears fills her eyes as her whole body judders.

'That should get a prize,' she says, barely getting the words out. 'It's alive!'

It's a laugh that makes me feel warm. No adult has made me feel that way since . . . when? Ever?

She sighs a long happy sigh and picks up her phone.

'Come on, I need to remember this.'

She turns it around and the battery warning flashes.

'Quick! The battery!'

Her voice is mock appalled, like she has just witnessed a terrible tragedy.

'Ohmigod, it feels like it's going to remove my heart. Please someone invent a phone that makes it through the day. Come on, I want that face on film.'

She squeezes herself onto my chair, presses her body against me and is warm and loose, and as she wraps one arm around me, I feel her breast against my side. I wrap both my arms around her and press my cheek to hers.

'I don't really like having my picture taken,' I say.

'Come on, just for us, just for memories.'

She pouts a bit, hamming it up for the camera, giving it trout lips, and raises the camera up, holding it as far away as she can and turning the lens to us. I am next to her and life feels good. She turns to me, tipsy, voice loud.

'Babes, this is the best night out I've had in months.'

And so I smile, and she clicks away.

'Now,' she says. 'It's way too late to go home. Let's have a sleepover. Noah goes in Scout's bed, you get the spare room. Then we can drink some more.'

And this place feels so warm and soft, and the wine buzzes in me so gently, that I smile and say, 'Yes.'

We take our tired children upstairs, both of them already drifting off. Lo gives me a spare pair of Scout's pyjamas for Noah, and we tuck them up. He has never had a sleepover before, and seeing him under a duvet, wrapped up with his best friend, fills my heart with warmth, makes me think that maybe he will be OK, that our lives might work.

Lo and I go downstairs and open one more bottle, settle on the sofa where the kids just sat, but we don't drink anything, both of us too drunk already.

'Oh, Lo, I'm battered. I hardly even drink now.'

'What! How do you get through the parenting day?'

'Umm, tea?'

'Tea!'

She is outraged. We sit back, say nothing, and she grips my left hand in both of hers and turns to look directly at me.

'Look,' she says, 'I know I'm pissed, but there's something I've been meaning to say, and I don't know how, so I'm just going to say it.'

She looks at me like she's about to propose.

'Dyl. I don't have the right words, and I don't expect you to say anything, but I've been thinking about your dad, and your partner, and how much tragedy you've lived through, losing them both . . .'

She pauses for a moment and just then I want to tell her: '*JD's not dead, he's just a very bad man and I wish he was.*'

'You don't have to say anything, Dyl, but I just want to say that it's shit. It's so shit. And I'm sorry that it's happened to you.'

She looks me in the eye and she means it and she cares, and just for a moment I want her to wrap around me. I want to put my head on her chest and feel her arms around my shoulders and hear her tell me things are getting better. But I don't know how to do that, so I just give her a little smile.

'Thanks, Lo. Thank you for everything.'

We're silent, and then I look away, down at my glass, and take another gulp.

An hour later, she leads me to her spare room. An entire bedroom: unneeded, set aside for guests. The small double bed is made, everything neat, all set up like a hotel.

'Ooh, look at you with your interiors.'

'Only the best, babes. Doesn't get much use, to be honest. Unless Johno is snoring. If he tries to get in with you, kick him.'

'OK.'

She stumbles out like that's it, goodnight, and I just stand there as she crashes about in her room across the landing.

Then she returns to present me with some dusty-pink paisley-silk pyjamas, neatly folded on her two upright hands.

'Your pyjamas, madam. These will be big for you, but you can wear them if you want.'

I take them and she throws herself at me in a long, deep hug.

'My love,' she says. 'It's been emotional.'

She kisses my forehead and stumbles away.

I stroke my hand over the bedspread, feel the pyjamas be-tween my fingers, undress and put them on. They feel soft on my skin, just drift across my limbs like they're part of me.

I am drunk and in her home.

In her clothes.

We have shown each other our fannies.

I guess this makes us friends.

21

DYLAN

The bed feels even better in the morning. It's like the duvet has grown softer and fatter in the dark. Like it has been healing me, and Lo's silk pyjamas have stroked my skin all night. It's a strange thing, sleeping in someone else's house, on a bed they once slept on, sheets they might have been in. It's like you're their family just for one night and they will look after you. You trust each other enough to close your eyes, and to see how each other looks first thing in the morning.

I pick up my phone and stab through my apps. On Instagram, @Wow!Now! loves her new platinum and rose gold earrings. I have another fifteen followers and a new DM from @hopingwaiting247.

'Thank you so much for your words. When it gets too dark, I read them again and again.'

Influenza reckons a woman I don't know has had collagen implants. It's an odd thing this site and you can barely follow a story, but I've found myself flicking back to it every now and then since Lo mentioned it.

On the news, Russians are hacking UK businesses. There are officially 4.5 million UK children living in poverty. Technically, that might include Noah.

It's 8.35 a.m.

Why isn't he awake?

I run out of the room and along the hall and fly into Scout's room and he's there, with her, playing with a little Lego family.

'Hey, Mummy.'

He gets up and hugs my leg, then goes back to his game.

'Hello, kids.'

'We're playing Lego,' says Noah.

'I can see.'

'This one's the mummy and this one's the daddy and these are the kids, but we can't find the dog.'

They turn back to their game. His words were a statement, not a call for help: 'This is what I'm doing, now you can move along.' I watch them in silence for a while, and then it feels intrusive. He is my child but this is not my house.

I feel weak, a little cold. Like I left the comfort of the bed too soon and my hangover wants to remind me that it's there.

I can hear a coffee machine whirring downstairs. Today would be a good day for coffee. I head down to see Lo.

I walk barefoot down their sanded wooden staircase, into the living room. It feels like living in an Instagram post. We were screaming drunk last night, but life today is soft and styled again.

As I get to the kitchen, I find Johno banging the coffee machine like it's an old tug-boat engine. He's in towelling shorts and a hoodie and smells of the morning. Like he woke up and pulled these things on and now I am here in his wife's silk pyjamas. I grip the loose sleeves with my fingers, hold them tight, so they don't ride up my arms.

'Hello,' he says, like an apology.

There's a faint whiff of booze on him and he looks pasty.

'Hiya, you all right?'

'Mmm. Had a works thing last night. Scout is not being sympathetic.'

'How long have they been up?'

'Since about six. Lo said it was my shift.'

'Oh, you should've woken me.'

'It's all right, no point us all suffering.'

'Was Noh OK?'

'Fine, very happy. I gave them snacks and juice and they ran around for a bit, jumped on me for a while, we watched some telly. I've been trying to convince them Lego might be fun for about two hours, and think we might now get about eight minutes' peace.'

'Well, thanks for looking after him.'

I don't think a man has ever played with Noah. Never been there for him to jump on.

'It's fine. Lo's in the shower. Do you want coffee?'

He's doing that thing that men sometimes do when they suck their cheeks in. He has his chin down towards his chest and his brows up, making his forehead wrinkle and his eyes all doleful, like he's Michael Bublé after the Grammys, rather than a suburban dad who's been experimenting with Jägerbombs.

We stand in the kitchen like teens at a party and the conversation pauses, because I've intruded in their life, caught him half naked.

Next to the coffee machine is a small cardboard crate full of tomatoes, with circus-style letters on the side that read: South Coast Toms Heritage Box. Some are bright red and fat as tennis balls, some glow yellow, others look more like grapes.

'You feeling a bit rough?'

ANNA WHITEHOUSE

'It was . . . a night.' He says this like I will understand.

'Well, at least you've got enough tomatoes.'

He laughs. 'They came this morning. We have a tomato subscription.'

He does the brow thing again, apologetically.

'I didn't know people could subscribe to tomatoes.'

'Me either.' He shrugs, tries to sparkle. 'They send us a box every month. Lo just does a post now and then. We wouldn't normally subscribe to tomatoes, I should be clear. Although they are delicious in salads.'

He plucks out one of the yellows and offers it to me. I take it and eat it and immediately want more.

'That really is delicious.'

It is sweet and juicy and I never knew toms could taste like that.

We move to their kitchen table, sipping coffee and picking at the smaller tomatoes straight from the box.

Johno's hoodie is zipped to three-quarters and I can see his clavicles and the top of his chest. There are little hairs there and I wonder what they're like together, him and Lo. Is the sex very slow and do they pose, or does he bang away like he did with the coffee machine?

I am suddenly starving and these toms are doing me good and just for a second this could be a life I lead, with nice food and a nice place and someone with me.

And then Lo arrives, bouncing into the room.

She's in a navy-linen jumpsuit and it moves easily but still makes out the shape of her body.

She has bigger breasts than me. She has more hips too. She's more womanly. She has more and is more in every way and my head aches and my stomach feels delicate.

She smiles.

200

'How are you feeling?'

I smile back.

'Been better. Haven't had a hangover in a long time. How about you?'

She reaches for a coffee cup and knocks it over, picks it up, places it under the spout of the machine.

'Yeah, not exactly camera-ready.'

She looks camera-ready. She looks perfect, ready to shine, ready to be photographed, but today her movements are clumsy. Sometimes I think she's very sophisticated, but then I think she's about to walk into a wall. She's like a beautiful cat chasing after a remote-control car.

She turns on the coffee machine, then turns to me again as it hums.

'Did you sleep OK?'

'Oh my God, really well. That bed is so comfortable.'

'Isn't it? I used to love it.'

'Were you up with the kids at six?'

'No, left that to this one.'

She nods at Johno, steps over, tousles his hair.

'Poor lamb didn't get in until three, stinking of fags.'

He shrugs, shrinks a little.

'Oh, wow.' I smile at him. 'You really took a hit for us.'

He tilts his head, smiles a gentle grin, self-deprecating but not.

'I'm really a very lovely man.'

Lo looks at him tenderly.

'Maybe we should let this one go. Your shift is done.'

His whole body loosens and a smile of relief expands across his face.

'Well thank chuff for that. I'd nearly run out of nice.'

There's a rumble of feet on the stairs, and the kids appear behind Lo. Noah has a wet stain across his pyjama bottoms.

'Mummy, I've had an accident,' he says.

'Oh, Noah.'

'Oh, dear,' says Lo.

'It's not wee,' says Scout, 'it's juice that Daddy gave us.'

'What happened, Noah Balboa? Were you working that left jab again?'

Johno does a mock punch in the air and Noah smiles awkwardly. A shared thing between them, from whatever games they've all been playing this morning.

'Sorry, Mummy,' says Noah, and for a minute I think he might cry.

'It's OK,' says Lo. 'Accidents happen.'

'Yes, I spilled it,' he says.

'And did you say sorry?' I ask.

'Sorry,' he says.

I feel inappropriate. Lo is dressed, clean, clothed. I am in nightwear with her husband and my boy is soiling her house. We should go.

'I'll wash it and bring it back,' I say.

'Oh, it's fine, don't worry,' says Lo.

'No, it's OK, I will.'

'Really, it's fine.'

Then Scout screams.

'Mummy, Noah can have some of the new clothes!'

'Yes! That's perfect!' She turns to me. 'We've got loads of stuff that will fit him.'

'It's fine, I've got his stuff from yesterday.'

'It's OK. A new batch came last week and it's never been worn. Most of it is kids wear and we've got way too much. Noah can just keep it.'

'We'll be like twins,' says Scout.

And Lo pulls out a big cardboard box from the cupboard under the stairs. It's stuffed full of jumpers and skirts and jeans and shorts and tees in pastel shades of green and yellow and beige, tags hanging off like stock for a new shop.

'It's this Swedish brand called Etisk. It's all ultra-ethical and recyclable and gender-neutral. There's sustainable wool and no microfibres.'

'What are microfibres?' asks Johno.

'I don't know, but there are none of them,' says Lo.

'They kill turtles,' I say.

And so she makes a careful selection of beige chinos, a green polo, a yellow cardigan. She hands me the clothes.

'Mummy,' says Scout. 'I'll wear mine too.'

So we change our children right there and suddenly my boy looks like a little man, even if that little man is a banker on a golfing holiday.

But he is also adorable.

'Noh, look at you! My little baby all grown up!'

He's colour matched to Scout and they look like they've fallen out of a Gap Kids catalogue.

'Oh my gosh, it's too much,' gasps Lo.

The kids look at each other.

'This is so cute,' says Lo. 'Let me get a picture.'

She squats down with her phone and takes a snap.

'I might crash out,' says Johno. 'This could take a while.'

He slopes away to lie in bed, and for a moment I'm just standing there, Lo's pyjamas loose and soft against my skin, as she poses our children.

'Just move back a little, kids,' she says, then taps the camera again.

She moves them around so their backs are against the wall,

shoots again. Scout flits into a smile, a practised, radiant grin. Noah stares, a little uncertain.

'Hey, guys,' says Lo, 'could you turn to each other and smile?'

They do, but Noah still looks unsure.

'Aw, that's lovely, guys,' I say. 'Now, do you want to play?'

'Hang on,' says Lo.

She's looking at her screen, silent, absorbed. She has our attention and we all pause like she's our director.

'OK, guys,' She says, her voice now alive, excited, a kids' TV presenter again.

She ushers them to the middle of the floor, lays them down on the floorboards, stands above them, flattens her phone, points it downward and my boy is a prop.

'Now, look at me, guys.'

She snaps some more and gives a tiny happy squeal.

'Oh my God, look at them, Dyl. Look at our children!'

She shows me the photo and it's my little man in his off-duty banker suit and her little girl in matching gear, lying back and holding hands. They are beaming true grins. My boy is happy, and it's an image I want to frame and keep forever.

'Etisk would LOVE this,' says Lo. 'You can even see the logo on his top.'

She looks at me like she's planning a bank raid.

'Oh my God, would you mind if I used it?'

'For what?'

'For an ad.'

'For what?'

'For Etisk. I have a deal with them. One post a month. This would be perfect.'

I just look at her.

'Look at your boy's beautiful face. We've got to make that famous.'

'But people will see.'

'Of course! But it's OK, they're all women. Like, ninety-seven per cent.'

But he's my boy, and I don't want people seeing him. I don't want JD seeing him. That face is mine.

But she just carries on.

'We'll split the fee: you could invoice me for two-hundred quid.'

She dishes it out like it's nothing: tissues, old sweet wrappers, £200. One quick snap and you've earned a month's food.

I think of the shabby cupboards back at the flat: the debts, the empty sales column on last week's ChatTeam.

'If this one goes well,' she says, 'maybe they could even do more?'

'What do you mean?'

'Scout and Noah: I need to do one of these posts a month and I'm running out of ideas to be honest. But two kids, that's lots more fun.'

'It's just so public.'

'Babes, you're a 'grammer now. You've got six-thousand followers.'

She's teasing, joking, but she's also pushing. I stay silent.

'It's OK,' she says. 'We don't have to. We'd just be helping each other out.'

She sounds insulted. Like I think what she does is wrong. Like it's beneath me. The kids are slowly getting up and if I just say yes, I get £200.

I don't even need to do anything, I just need to say yes to this woman who is trying to help me. Then the debt people go away for a month, or the cupboards get properly filled.

She helped me with Noah's project, and she's helped him

make friends with her daughter and she's helped people see my words.

'Maybe,' she says, 'we could try this one, split the fee, and if you're comfortable, we do this every month.'

'Every month?'

'Yeah, it's easy money, really.'

'But couldn't we do it again, with his face turned away?'

She shakes her head slowly, like this is impossible.

'It's the eye contact with the lens. People really respond to eye contact. The algorithm, too.'

She just needs me to help her.

'All I need is to borrow that adorable face,' she says.

How bad can it be if she does it with her own kid?

'But you never know who will see it,' I say.

'It's just mums. And they forget as soon as their scrolling finger moves on.'

JD's not going to be following posh mums on Instagram.

'I do it with Scout all the time and have never had a problem.'

He hasn't even seen Noah. Wouldn't even recognise him.

'OK, let's do it.'

'Oh, amazing, this is such a help, thanks, Dyl.'

She looks genuine. Like she's relieved and grateful. I have helped her and she has helped me.

'It'll be fine,' she says. 'It's just for mums like us. Now, we've got a playdate to get to.'

'Oh, yeah,' says Scout, beaming, excited, 'with Martha!'

Noah's face grows still.

'A friend from nursery,' Lo says. 'We haven't seen her in ages, have we, Scout?'

'No!'

And I can see in Noah's face something that I feel, too. A little burn in the belly. They have other friendships that don't involve us. Because that's normal. People are supposed to have more than one friend.

Lo turns to me.

'Do you want a shower?'

I stand under the shower they both use, my body warm and naked where theirs go every day. I use her soaps, her scented scrubs, Clinique and Molton Brown. It's an odd thing, to use someone else's shower. Like you're doing something indecent in their home. Then I dry myself, dress, dab water splashes off the floor with the towel she has lent me.

I go downstairs and we get our shoes on, and as our children hug, Lo wraps herself around me, pulls me tight to her, presses her breasts against mine, her arms around me.

'Oh my God, that was such fun. We should do this again, soon.'

'Definitely,' I tell her.

And with my hair still wet, we step out of this little holiday in her life, with its comfort and softness and warmth, ushered out like a one-night stand and sent home.

22

LO

The pregnancy test is tucked in the inside pocket of my bomber jacket, along with crumpled receipts and chewing gum. I bought it from a pharmacy by the Tube because I need to know, but now I'm running late, so I start jogging along Dewant Mews, a cul-de-sac of calm in the middle of Soho. My bag is tightly clamped under my arm and I focus on the grey paving slabs that lock London together.

Jenn asked me in for a quick meeting before the panel with the big insurance firm, Allegiance. Somewhere in between, I will find a loo and hope for that blue cross to emerge through the urine-soaked cotton. A little verification for my hostile uterus. A blue tick for motherhood. My boobs hurt and my stomach is bloated, but I can't let myself think it's someone yet.

I get to Dewant House and the automatic glass doors open sharply. As I walk in, a man wearing a denim jumpsuit and box-fresh trainers strides out. He looks familiar even though I've never met him before. The scent of aftershave lingers in his wake and he's being pursued by a small Pomeranian dog on a lead.

'Who are you here to see?' says Den, the receptionist, who

doubles as a security guard. He's got eyes like chestnuts and his face is set to a permanent grin. He's older, sixty maybe, but with the energy of a bartender at happy hour.

'Jenn, on the twelfth floor.'

'Are you talent?' he says, giving me a wry smile, which defuses the awkwardness of answering that question.

'Yes,' I say, wondering what exactly my talent is. I tap a screen and spill my mind and somehow that earns money.

He gives me a friendly wink and the barrier opens abruptly. Just behind his glass desk is a photo of him hugging a woman who mirrors his smile and I wonder if they are as happy as they look. He has a 'Give Blood' pin on his left lapel, and he waves me into the building like it's my first day of school.

The lift smells of aftershave and stale air, like the fragrance section in a department store. I press '12' and it jolts into action as I stare at my face in the mirror. Mascara has smudged onto my upper lid and I rub it too hard with my index finger, leaving a red mark in place of a black one. I don't recognise myself, even though I've been seen today by 64,000 strangers. Creases under my eyes are weighed with foundation that makes them look like dusty ravines. I run my fingers back through my hair to try to give it some lift, and strands come away and float to the ground. My floral tea dress pops in pink and green and accentuates my slightly creped breasts and I regret wearing it.

The lift doors open and I breathe in, happy to be in a grown-up space instead of surrounded by Weetabix and dirty school uniforms. Everything smells of rose water here, instead of a rotting packed-lunch box. There are fifty white desks, most with beautiful twenty-five-year-old women staring intently at MacBooks. Some look ready for cocktails or photo shoots. I can never bring Johno here. He wouldn't know where to look.

HMN Hub has a big neon sign above its entrance that reads:

'Kindness Costs Nothing' – and I wonder how that works when someone is made redundant.

Maybe I should do the pregnancy test now, get it over with before settling down with Jenn. I go to walk to the toilets, hand pressing down on the test in my pocket, butterflies in my stomach like I'm about to have a job interview.

'LO!'

Jenn interrupts, strides towards me, arms outstretched.

'So good to see you, my love. How's it going? I mean, big question, I know,' she laughs, her red bra showing through her cream silk top. Her eyebrows look like someone has taken a marker pen to them. Like a beautiful Angry Bird. 'Ignore the brows,' she says, waving dismissively at her forehead. 'They've just been done but will calm down in a day or so. Why don't you get yours sorted while we chat?'

She gestures towards a makeshift brow bar in the corner of the office and before I can consider if I want to look permanently furious, I'm sitting down in front of a woman called Suze who is wielding a miniature paintbrush. Jenn is standing by my side, a hand draped across my shoulder. I consider asking to go to the toilet, like a toddler at nursery, but before I can move, two huge breasts are in my face.

'So what are we doing?' asks Suze, scanning my face for something that's missing. She's wearing an apron with a logo on it – 'Raised Brows' – and I can't decide if that's an appalling name or not. She smells of cigarettes and spearmint.

'I'll just have a tidy-up, if that's OK?' I tell her.

'You want a light tint? You will barely notice it?'

She begins to prepare one.

'Do it, Lo,' says Jenn. 'Honestly, you won't regret it. I was wary at first.'

'No, I'm OK, thanks.'

I close my eyes and sink into the seat. The brash, office light pushes through my lids and my thoughts flash back to Lina and the moment they told her that Oscar had no heartbeat.

'Lo, I've seen the first shots from the WeAreFemForm shoot. Dang, girl, you look hot,' says Jenn.

'I thought I looked like a pantomime dame,' I say quietly, absorbing the pinches of Suze's plucking.

'No, love, you looked gawj.'

'Good. It was a bit of a surprise about the experiment, to be honest.'

'Oh, I know, but they said you handled it brilliantly.'

Suze tilts my head to reach a stubborn hair between my brows.

'I should have known before going, though. I was really on the spot.'

'I know, love. Honestly, their briefings are so sketchy.'

'So they didn't tell you?'

'They're really disorganised. But what's great is they want to use the images of you across all networks. They said you were so real, so honest, and it means we can charge more. You happy to go ahead?'

My left eyebrow is burning slightly and Suze's elbow is resting on my forehead and I gently give a go-ahead 'Mm-hmm'.

Jenn's ignored my question, though. I don't believe they didn't tell her about the experiment, but I need her on side. I need her bringing the deals in. I'm her client, but she is also, in a way, my boss and the one who gets me paid.

Suze is sweeping my brows with a soothing, cold liquid. Then she holds up a mirror for me and my brows look as though they've been stuck on like fridge magnets.

'Thank you, I love them.'

Jenn gasps. 'They're perfect!'

I've always liked Jenn, but I wonder if she'd prefer to be on my side of the smartphone: a face rather than a fixer.

I stand up as Suze realigns her kit, waiting for her next subject.

'Thanks so much.'

'You're welcome. A strong brow really suits you.'

'Thanks. It's great.'

She doesn't believe that I'm convinced.

'It'll settle in two days, then you need a touch-up every month. I'm here every first Tuesday. It's a company perk.'

'Great, thanks. It's lovely.'

Jenn returns with a glass of water and leads me to a side office with glass walls, overlooked by a bank of white desks. The walls have thin black strips running horizontally and vertically, so every space of the room is within a square black frame. Inside is a large, bright-red armchair that Jenn takes, and a brown leather one for me, with a cow-print rug between them.

'Now, love, there's something I need to talk to you about, and while you are in town for your panel, I thought it'd be good to do it face to face.'

She's adopted the serious expression of a person about to break up with someone.

'It's about your engagement. It's really going down quite quickly now.'

She's a few years younger than me, but is smiling and nodding with the encouraging face of a nursery-school teacher.

'But I've been picking up loads of followers,' I say.

'I know, and that's great,' she says. 'But it's engagement that brands look at: how many of your followers are liking your stuff, and that has really fallen away. It's totally, totally normal. We manage Jabba the Mutt and he saw a massive drop in engagement when he did an ad for a dog-walking service called Doggie Style.'

She laughs, flicking to her phone like it's an extension of her hand, and I do the same. The meeting pauses for a moment, as we both stare at a slobbering British bulldog wearing a miniature fuchsia-pink 'Doggie Style' T-shirt.

Jenn snaps back to business.

'But you just need to keep posting, like we said. Once a day as a basic to feed the algorithm. Though twice would be amazing.'

'Do you think the dog knows?'

'Knows what?'

'That he's being sold on the internet?'

'I mean, he doesn't seem that bothered.' She leans forward and holds my gaze. 'And besides, he'll be billing 250k a year, and that's a lot of doggie treats.'

She's telling me I'm being outshone by a canine.

'We just need to make sure you're doing as well as you can be. People don't mind the ads if you're giving them enough organic content. Just think about what more you could put out there.'

She smiles, so I do.

'OK, great, thanks for the tip.'

Jenn stands up and smooths down her yellow silk skirt, indicating the meeting is over. She leads the way out of the office and as we stride towards the main door, her willowy figure cuts through the office, the way you can when armed with youth. She pecks my cheek as she says goodbye.

'Good luck today. You're gonna nail it.'

I kiss her cheek, walk out and head straight to the toilet.

The door of the powder-pink cubicle swings shut and I lock it and sit on the toilet seat. I stare ahead at an advert for hair-loss supplements that starts: 'At a hair loss?' which makes no sense.

I put my phone on the top of a metal toilet-roll holder above the sanitary bin. There's the blue plastic of a tampon applicator poking out of the lid. I tap my chest and feel the pregnancy test jut into my ribcage.

Now is the moment.

I hold on to my wee and unwrap the pregnancy test. I have learned through experience that trying to catch the first flow just leaves you with wet fingers, so I hover over the seat.

It's beginning to feel like my major life moments all happen on the toilet. My first ad was for bog roll, my last miscarriage was on the toilet at daycare. And now, another pregnancy test.

I've done so many that the blue line feels more like a warning than a celebration: *disappointment lies ahead. Not this time, maybe try again. Do not pass GO, your uterus is still hostile.*

I pee on the stick, a little urine splashing off the plastic onto my hand. How long do we keep trying when it's stopping us from living?

I stare at the test, willing it to answer straight away, then pull up my knickers, stand and turn to my phone to calm the buzz in my head.

Amara has messaged.

'My love. The Influenzans are kicking OFF. Lots about you I'm afraid. Just thought you should know. Always here. X'

She's included links. The familiar magenta-and-grey palette stares back at me. My hands go cold. I stand still next to the hand dryer, setting it off slightly, jumping backwards, my phone in one hand, the pregnancy test limply in the other.

The title reads: 'How much is a child worth?'

Someone has photoshopped my face onto the Virgin Mary's and Scout's onto Jesus's. Scout has a dollar sign scribbled across her face. I hold my breath and feel my lungs compress. Anger floods my body, my cheeks feel numb and heat pulses to my face. Who uses the face of an innocent child to make a point?

I glance at the pregnancy test, but the urine hasn't fully soaked through. I flick back to the thread. It's too hot in this airless cubicle. It's a lightless box.

> **Floggetyflog says:** I don't buy this worthier-than-thou bullshit. She's using 'the patriarchy' to hide the fact she's flogging her child online. I know Scout and she doesn't know me. If that doesn't chill you as a mother . . .

There are 156 responses already and my heart starts to thump.

> **SweetCaroline says:** Can you imagine being able to put a price on your child's privacy? My mate works with her and she got £10,000 for that Etisk stuff. It's like a black comedy. These women have no idea what they're actually selling. Scout has been served up to paedophiles. What mother puts a price on innocence?

What does she mean paedophiles? What paedophiles? And how do they know about the money? Only people here know about the money. Or at WeAreFemForm.

I feel the heat pushing into my chest as I look at the test. It's not been three minutes.

I go back to the thread, sink further in. New comments keep popping up and it keeps moving, strangers united by their objection to me.

> **OhFlogOff says:** Can you imagine Scout googling her mother and finding this thread? All those forced happy-family moments given

215

away to strangers.

SweetCaroline says: She'll hate her when she's older.

OhFlogOff says: She's got every right to.

JaneOfTheJungle says: Does anyone know who that other kid is? The little boy in her last ad? Bet his mum wants to cash in too if she's from the same 'Girl Gang'.

I accidentally set off the hand dryer again with my elbow and jump at the sound, hitting my elbow against the wall. There are 198 comments now, and 8,456 people are viewing the thread.

But who are these women?

Why do they hate me?

How do they know what I earn?

I flush the toilet, diluting the dark amber of my urine and stare into the mirror. I look like my make-up has been painted on. Like I'm wearing a Venetian mask, the thick, clay paint unable to hide the grey of my skin.

I wave the stick as tears burn.

Maybe I *am* exploiting Scout.

Maybe I *am* annoying.

Maybe I *am* fake.

But I'm also pregnant.

A blue cross.

I hold tears back, blink them right back, pull the air inside myself and breathe out slowly. Roll back my shoulders, chin up.

I need to work.

23

DYLAN

ChatTeam is open, but I flick to my phone. I'm like some stock trader, double screening: when I pause from Big Work internet, Little Phone internet is right there, with my gang of 7,412.

These numbers are mad. It's not Lo's scale, but it's still mad. People keep saying how much I'm helping them, how much they love my words.

@wangtg
Ohmigod, the school photos! I've got a camera on my phone and I see their faces every day! Why you tryn to guilt me!

People are tired of the polish. They want some truth.

I spin again and there's a new DM, from @hopingwaiting247.

'I just made pommes de terre de toms! I loved it!'

Then I flick to Lo's feed and scroll down to Noah's face, and I can't stop looking at it.

My boy and her girl, smiling for the camera, 200 comments,

a few thousand likes. People are saying how cute they are together. And they are. They are adorable.

But what about the ones who don't like it? There must be hundreds scrolling by, thousands maybe. Sighing or tutting, feeling nothing and scrolling on, and I wonder where they are and what they're doing. People are looking at him while sitting on the bog, or the bus, at work, eating crisps on the sofa.

Something precious and perfect that I know so well, taken and repackaged and held up for others to judge, just to give them a microsecond of warmth, just enough to nudge their thumb down fractions of a millimetre to tap. Or them seeing it and hating it and thinking he's a dick. She's creating micro-feelings for strangers, and using my boy's face to do it.

I've been feeling a little sick since it went up. Like I've given away something sacred and can't get it back. This is what it means to earn money this way, I guess, and maybe it's not worth it.

But she's already paid me and some of it's spent and sitting in the fridge and the cupboard.

Maybe I just shouldn't do any more after this one.

ChatTeam glows, but it can wait. It's good to have breaks.

I cycle through the news and check my emails.

Dear Dylan,

The Women Who Watch On

Many thanks for submitting your proposal for your novel *The Women Who Watch On.* We think it is a wonderful idea and addresses some important issues that are too often ignored. We have been following your work on social media, and think you offer a vibrant and engaging new voice on a subject in desperate need of illumination. We'd be delighted to discuss the proposal in more detail. Would you be able to come to our offices in Norwich?

Yours

Callum Colquhoun
Publisher
Recondite Books

I close the email and open it again.

The words feel foreign and my phone feels light in my hand.

I read it and close it and open it again: 'wonderful idea . . . engaging new voice . . . discuss the proposal'.

I look up and around the flat. The little table where Noah sat this morning, scraping up the last spoonful of porridge. I look around the room – this tired room, with its tired furniture and greying walls and its chipped, scuffed, scabby little surfaces. I look for someone to share this with and, of course, there's no one here.

But someone wants me.

Wants my words and my ideas.

Someone thinks I have something to say and that I can say it well.

Maybe even enough to pay me.

I feel a little tear creep to the corner of my eye.

And then I laugh. A short little 'Ha!' just leaps out of me and I turn my phone down with a slam because I can't believe it. My cheeks feel warm and a smile bursts across my face.

I'm like some mad woman laughing in a dingy little kitchen all on her own.

I just stand for a while, and wonder what this might mean.

It means I have to go to Norwich.

I flick to trainline.com. It's two hours by train. I can drop Noah off and be back for pick-up.

Sixty quid each way!

No, wait, ha! That's tomorrow. Super advanced is £20 return. Still, £20 though. And a month's wait. What if he doesn't still want it in a month? I tap at my phone.

Dear Callum,

This is delightful news. Many thanks for considering me. I am free for a call or video chat? Travel is difficult with the school run.

Warm regards,

Dylan Rayne

Send.

I stand there and wait like he's going to reply straight back. I just stare at my phone screen, waiting for something to pop into the inbox. Refresh, nothing. Refresh, nothing. I shouldn't have said the bit about the school run. It makes me sound lame. Like I'm some mum banging things out around the washing. I mean, I am that, but I shouldn't look like it.

Of course! How inconsiderate of me. I'm actually in London in a couple of weeks. Could we meet then? A quick lunch on us?

Cal

HA!

It comes out like a firework pop.

It's fine.

It's fine, Dyl.

There's a tingle all over me. These wonderful charges running around my limbs like my blood is fizzing.

My life is changing so fast.
Yes, I would love to have a quick lunch, Cal.
More than anything.
More than any single thing I have ever done.

24

LO

I step out of the building, autumn whips my face and I huddle into my jacket and lock my hands around my phone. The pregnancy test is still in my pocket, evidence that cells are forming, even if they might suddenly stop one day. My mind keeps trying to imagine the person growing, but my heart won't let me add detail.

I walk slowly and swipe across from Instagram's red hearts and flick to Influenza. Scout's face gazes out from my home screen and then the magenta page starts to load. I type 'Lo' and 'Down' into the search icon and step into a doorway that smells of urine, a steady flow of Londoners passing me by. There's a small sticker peeling off one of the tiles that says, 'free hugs', but doesn't say where. I hold one hand to my face, enjoying the stillness for a second and with the other click on the thread again. They've changed the name to 'Lo: The Mother of All Cunts'. There are 235 responses now.

Floggetyflog says: I don't know what I struggle with more, her or the sheep that bleat about 'how brave' she is sitting there, flashing her tits. Imagine a postnatally-depressed, vulnerable mother following her and lapping up her waffle about flashing your nips and then next post she's flogging them a £200 breast pump as an 'essential item'.

But I've never done a breast-pump ad. You can't just say, 'imagine' and make something true!

Loveisallaround says: I don't think this thread should be called 'Mother of all cunts', because what's so bad about a vagina? We need to stop using women's genitals to slate people we can't stand. And let's be clear, I cannot stand Lo Knox.

Blahblahblah says: My sister works with her husband and he's very 'handsy'. Funny how they put out this whole 'couple goals' shit and he's snogging the intern in the bogs.

My eyes prickle.

Is he?

Is my husband 'handsy'?

Maybe he was, with me, at the beginning. A little squeeze when no one was looking. But not for a while. Not now.

Now it's a peck on the cheek to say hello, a dab of lips to say goodbye, a tired fumble after watching documentaries about women who kill.

So he's snogging the intern in the bogs while I'm pregnant with his child.

He mentioned a new girl. Eilis. She 'can't add up'. He joked that none of her clothes fit. That her sleeves stopped at the elbows and her trousers at the calf.

She'll be young. Probably doesn't have a stomach that pools to one side when she turns over in bed. Jesus, Johno.

Something crashes into my back and I squeal as my phone flies to the floor. A pitiful little sound. A guy in tight black

223

jeans squeezes out of the door, huffs and is absorbed by the crowd.

I reach down and pick up my phone. The screen is a black, cracked mirror. Everything is on there. My banking, my writing, my life and my livelihood. I need to know what's being said, I need to call Johno, I need to know the time and where I'm going.

I rub it gently on my palm to remove a wet leaf. Tiny shards of glass catch my skin and I swipe softly, moving next to an abandoned phone box decked with escort business cards. There's a woman whose breasts have 'free hugs' stickers on them. Someone else pushes past me like I'm an obstacle.

I can just about see the time. And where I need to get to.

The Allegiance building is five minutes from Canary Wharf station. It is tall and glass and towers over other buildings, like it's a competition of girth and length. The lobby is full of people, mostly men, frowning into phones as they walk.

The receptionist smiles at me without giving any sense of who is behind that smile. The desk is long and wood-panelled, hinting at something oddly traditional in this very modern space.

'Who are you here for?'

'I'm here for the Allegiance panel event.'

'Do you know what department?'

'No, I know it starts at 2.00 p.m.'

'OK, it's five minutes to two.'

'Yes. Is it David McAllister?'

I very gently swipe the surface of my phone like it's a precious gem. There's a flicker of movement and my heart leaps. I swipe again, across to the calendar, catching tiny grains of glass in my thumb but swiping on.

It pops up and I shout, 'It is David McAllister!'

She looks at me like I'm a kid that's been let loose in her father's office. But then her smile returns, and she taps at her keyboard.

'Here's your pass, the lifts are on the left; it's on the eighteenth floor.'

She turns her attention to the woman behind me.

I get in the lift with a crowd of people wearing grey or black in varying cuts. I look in the mirrored wall and my hair has been flattened by the London air and I look pale against my floral tea dress.

Johno wouldn't have an affair.

He's many things, but he's not a liar. He couldn't sleep with me and sleep with her. Whoever she is. He wouldn't do that.

I look up at the mirrored ceiling of the lift and look down on myself and I don't fit in. These are not work colours; I'm dressed like an eccentric. These aren't clothes that mean business. There is a light mascara stain on my lapel and I try to rub it off, smudging it further into the fabric. I look at my stomach, slightly bloated with life, and try not to wonder who he or she is.

The lift stops at every floor and I feel my phone in my pocket and get it out, my reflection distorted in the cracked screen. I need to find a toilet, to sweep some colour into my face and wrap something around the tiny red dots of blood on my thumb.

At the eighteenth floor, I step out alone and a woman in a grey trouser suit is waiting.

'You must be Lo!'

She says this in a way that suggests she is surprised to see me.

'Yes, so sorry I'm late, there was a bit of—'

'Come this way,' she says, skimming over my excuses and gently touching my lower back.

'Do I have time to go to the toilet?'

'David is just about to do his opening remarks. I'm so sorry, do you think you can hang on for half an hour? You were a little later than we expected.'

She smiles emptily.

'Sure, no problem.'

I suck the tip of my thumb, a tingle of salt rushing to the roof of my mouth.

Outside the conference room is a sign that reads: '(Wo)man up: an entry to allyship'.

She leads me into the room. There are fifty chairs set up lecture-style, most of them filled with men in suits. David is sitting on a raised stool at the front of the room, with two women on stools to his left and a third for me. He smiles at me and nods. I smile back and perch on the seat.

'Right,' he says, addressing the room.

The murmuring settles and conversations fall silent as everyone looks towards him.

'Let me start with introductions.'

He looks round at us and smiles, then clicks the clicker in his palm. On the screen behind and above us, my face appears. It's an image from my Instagram feed. I am face-on to the camera, standing with my legs planted widely, my arms raised and both biceps curled up like a vintage bodybuilder. Scout is in front of me, striking the same pose.

What was Johno thinking as he took that photo? Was he thinking of her? Of his new girl.

'Starting from the left, we have Insta-activist, Lo Knox.'

The room looks at me in silence. The fifty faces in the audience, the three to my right on the panel.

I smile a broad smile and give a little wave.

'Hi!'

I am pregnant.

My husband is having an affair.

Paedophiles have pictures of my daughter.

Thousands of women despise me.

And the worst part – the part that makes me want to run from this room – is that, from the things they're saying, and the details they know, these aren't all just strangers. These aren't trolls in dark basements. Some are women I've met, worked with, maybe even smiled at and shaken hands with.

These must be women who know me.

25

DYLAN

Noah is eating a chocolate biscuit in the bath because we're celebrating. I'm sitting by the tub, and he's smiling like it's Christmas. Chocolate is for Fridays, but today is a school night and he looks at me like he has discovered a new world.

He's cross-legged and munching his Penguin bar, little crumbs falling in the water, and his face says he never realised life could be this good. Maybe I didn't either.

Today, no bills came, but an email did and someone wants to take me out to lunch and talk about my book. It's like a thing that happens to other people. A day of firsts for both of us.

There are fish and chips keeping warm in the oven. In the chippy, Noah pressed his face to the glass of the fridge and I got him a Capri Sun, even though we'd got squash at home. Once he's ready, we will munch it all like gluttons and bollocks to the cost. Then snakes and ladders before bed.

I watch him as he eats the last bite of his Penguin, then hands me the wrapper.

'Was that good?'

'Yeah.'

228

The crumbs have all sunk to the bottom of the water, and it's time to get out. I hoist him up, wrap a towel around him, binding up his arms so just his head peeks out.

'I'm gonna wrap you up like a spring roll.'

I squeeze around him and he giggles as I rub my hands over the towel, keeping him warm, making him dry. There's a draught from the window here, so I always work fast. He goes limp and lets me carry him in my arms like a baby.

'Special delivery for Noah's room!'

I stand him up and pull his pyjamas out from under his pillow. He's normally a bit ratty by this stage, pushing me off, wanting to play with toys instead of getting ready for dinner and bed, but eating a Penguin in the bath has revealed a magical new world to him.

'Mummy, are the fish and chips for me too?'

'Of course, Noh! I'm not going to eat them on my own.'

'I thought the Penguin was my dinner.'

'No, the Penguin was a treat.'

'Because I'm good?'

'Yes, Noh, you're good.'

'Because I was good with Scout's mummy?'

'When, Noh?'

'When she made us take pictures.'

'Yes, Noh.'

He goes quiet and I slip his pyjama trousers over his legs, button up the top. It never occurred to me what it might feel like for him, being posed like that, made to perform.

'Did you like it, Noah, having your picture taken?'

He shrugs, turns his lips down.

'Yeah.'

He's casual, but I'm not sure.

'It's OK if you didn't.'

He shrugs again, either bored or traumatised – and with kids, you never really know which.

'All right,' I say, 'how about those fish and chips?'

He nods and smiles and we go through to the kitchen. I pull the food from the oven, unwrap the plain white paper, slide our portions onto plates, add a big dollop of ketchup and take the plates to the table.

I watch him as his little fingers press into the fat chips and he grins as he chews. I break off the end of my cod, the batter snapping as bits flake loose, and pick but don't really eat. I smile at Noah, and he looks at me, those blue eyes deep as a well, then he looks down, shy for a second, like I've been staring too long.

'Is it good?'

He nods, says 'Mm-hmm,' because chips are better than words.

I pick up my phone, flick to Instagram and Lo's feed, scroll back to the picture of our kids together.

He does look happy there, this version of him and Scout like beautiful siblings. There are more likes now, more comments too. I look to the top of the list, and a new one appears.

@Motherofdingbat$
You just ignoring the fact that you're getting ten grand from Etisk to flog your kid's face?

I stop and read it again, and another comment appears.

@Of{Course}SheDid
Yes, because she's shameless!

She got ten grand for Etisk? How do they know? That can't be right. Maybe that's for the whole year or something.

I mean, it's fine, if it is. Good luck to her.

And I said yes.

I accepted her money and I needed it.

But ten grand for her kid, and her nice house, and my share's a little bit of change on the side?

I look at Noah as he dry-gulps another chip.

'Silly me,' I say. 'I didn't get us any drinks!'

I walk over to the counter, pull some squash from the cupboard, put a little in one of his plastic cups and top up with water.

I walk back, give Noah his drink, stroke his hair and sit down; but I can't eat, because I need to see that picture again.

It is something so perfect, that picture. A tiny capsule of time shared between my son and his friend. And now it has been taken and served to others for a few pixels of entertainment.

A moment in his life as a tool to pause thumbs.

And she got ten grand, and we got £200.

While Noah eats, I tap out a message.

'Hey Lo! How are you? I wondered if I could talk to you about that post of Noah? X'

I watch my phone, as though Lo might reply straight away.

But she doesn't, of course.

She must get lots of messages.

26
LO

Johno opens the door with a wide grin. The smell of Bolognese wafts from the kitchen and I can see Scout sitting in the lounge playing with Lego. Jazz is trickling from the speakers. Scout spots me and thunders over, wrapping her small body around my leg.

'How was your day?' asks Johno, as Scout scampers back to her multicoloured construction, singing to herself, 'Mummy's home.'

'I broke my phone,' I say.

'Oh, no, that's annoying.'

And I am pregnant, and you're having an affair.

The table is set and there's the head of a single red rose from the garden in a clay ramekin. He hasn't ever set the table like this before.

He's moving around the kitchen, stirring the sauce, clattering around in a cupboard as he tries to prise Scout's favourite elephant plate from under a tower of Tupperware. It's like crockery Jenga.

'How did it break?'

'It's not completely broken, just the screen a bit.'

I want to ask him about the girl. I want to clear the anger rising in my chest. But Scout is here and I don't know if I can hold back once I start.

He lays knives and forks on the table with the precision of a silver-service waiter, using his fingertips to line up the edges, very precise and delicate.

Where else have those hands been?

What parts of her have they touched?

Did he make the first move, or did she?

Was it afterwork drinks, standing too close to each other as they shared a cigarette?

'I got us some nice wine from the corner shop. The nine-quid bottle, not the six-quid. Proper fancy.'

He smirks to himself. I can't look at him so I look at the floor and stare at a small crack on one of the tiles.

'I'm pregnant. I found out today.'

It comes out of nowhere and I let the news hang in the air and don't look at him. Anger rises in my throat. I don't want him to hug me or kiss me or touch me. I just want him to absorb the information so I can see how he reacts.

He straightens up, a smile fills his face. He looks delighted, like a toddler that's just won a stuffed toy on Brighton Pier.

I want to ask him if he's been whispering into the intern's ear as I grow his child.

But his exuberance throws me off.

Before I can do anything, he's wrapped me up in his arms and we're hugging. He steps back, surveys my stomach like the proudest man on earth, and for a fleeting moment I feel safe.

Either he's a liar, or they are.

I still have my coat on. He takes it off for me and comes back to give me another squeeze, this time grabbing both my bum cheeks like he's sizing up pumpkins. He looks into my eyes, searching them, picking up my reluctance.

'I know it's early, but we can give ourselves this moment,' he says.

'It is good news,' I say.

'It is good news.'

We stand in silence for a few seconds, trying to let some light in as I survey the dinner set-up.

'What's all this for?' I ask.

He looks genuinely happy, but there's a prolonged silence.

'I also have some news,' he says, smiling at me.

Johno never has news.

'I quit. I quit my job.'

He beams, like we've just got engaged.

I go limp, processing the information and his glee and wondering whether or not he has told another woman what he wants to do to her.

'What do you mean, you quit?'

I'm holding onto the cold-marble kitchen countertop, remaining neutral as best I can.

He goes back to stirring the sauce and turns his back on me.

'I didn't get Assistant Finance Director. I've been doing the job for six months, basically. All the extra work since Kwame moved up, all the responsibility and stress, but without the extra money or title.'

'You quit without talking to me?'

He stops stirring and looks at me.

'Lo, they didn't even tell me. I read it on a company-wide email. "A big welcome to yada yada." So, I quit. I'm going solo. What do you think of "Knox Finance"? Sounds a bit like Fort Knox in the States.'

I just stare at him.

'Or maybe "Pay the Fiddler"? I'll be offering niche accounting services to the music and entertainment industries.'

'Why? When did you decide this?'

My voice cracks slightly and my hands clench the counter. I can feel the day's pressure building in my chest and warming the back of my throat. He goes back to stirring.

'I decided today, but I've been thinking about it for a while. I've been there six years; they've been taking me for granted. Your social stuff is going well. It just felt the right time.'

'Why didn't you talk to me?'

I can feel my voice getting louder. My hand rests on my belly.

'Well, you've been a bit distracted and I didn't want to add to your stress.'

'This is adding to my stress!'

Shouting won't help, but he makes me want to shout. He's just so casual, so breezy, and I don't know if he's lying.

He puts down the wooden spoon and just seems to sigh a tiny bit, then he turns round and opens his arms for an embrace, but I turn away.

'This is an exciting moment. This is a good thing. We will both be running our own businesses. That's the only way to make any proper money.'

'But you're not making any money. You haven't got any clients. What about notice? Don't you have to give them a month's notice?'

'A clean break's best. I don't want to hang around; they don't want me there with all their sensitive information.'

'But you're not a rival. They're not an accountancy firm.'

He hesitates. 'It's just cleaner.'

'But why? You could have another month's salary. You could have another month to find clients.'

'Honestly, Lo, it's just cleaner. This isn't an ending, it's a beginning.'

He sounds like a slogan cushion. This isn't him. I'm pregnant and now I'm the sole breadwinner.

'What really happened, Johno? What happened that means you can't go back?'

'Well, I quit, Lo. When you quit, you have to leave.'

He's talking like I'm an imbecile.

'But why did you quit?'

'I've just told you, Lo! Jesus, I knew you wouldn't get it, but I just thought . . .' He stands back, deflated. '. . . I just thought that maybe you'd be with me. Two years ago, you'd have been with me. You'd have been excited. You'd be saying, "yeah, do it". I just thought . . .'

'Thought what?'

'I just thought there might be some of that left.'

'Some of what?'

'The old Lo.'

It just sits in the air. This is my fault, he's saying. He can quit his job of six years on a whim, and I'm some sour-faced shrew for questioning it.

Old Lo was fun and gave great blow jobs and made perfect poached eggs, but she's not me anymore so he has to quit work and take a mistress, and resentful New Lo is to blame.

'Well, maybe the old Johno wouldn't have touched up the intern.'

He straightens his back, rolls his shoulders and flexes his brow. He's trying to look bewildered. But what follows is scorn.

'What?' His eyes have gone dead and his brows have angled down. He's almost sneering. 'What are you saying?'

He goes to shut the kitchen door, but it's too late, Scout appears, in the way kids always do when an atmosphere darkens.

'Scouty, go and play with your Lego,' he says, sounding slightly desperate.

'Why are you and Mummy shouting?'

Johno scoops her up, takes her back to the sofa and turns on the TV. She looks so small and alone on those fat cushions.

'Sometimes grown-ups just need to talk about things, that's all,' he tells her. He skims channels, stops at the first kids' show he finds and strides back to the kitchen.

His eyes are wild and he gently shuts the kitchen door before removing the Bolognese from the heat and then turning to me.

'What did you just say? About an intern?'

I can't decide if he looks terrified or furious.

'It doesn't matter. Let's talk about it later.'

'Lo, you can't just drop that and then say we'll talk about it later. Are you insinuating I have had an affair? Is that where we are? Because if so, it does matter.'

He looks me directly in the eye and it makes me shrink backwards. The silence is barbed and I stare at the tiles on the floor. I need to get online. I need to know what else they're saying. But I also need him to speak.

'OK. Fine, we can do this now. Are you having an affair?'

I square up to him and watch.

'NO. No I'm not. Where did that even come from?'

He's angry. He's scornful. He's looking at me in a way I don't like. His face has become unfamiliar.

'I quit my job, Lo, because I am so utterly, wholly miserable. I expected you to be concerned, but not this. When did you stop being on my side?'

I wince at his words.

He runs his hands through his hair and leans against the sink. The Bolognese has a glistening film across it like the first morning frost. Johno looks up, his face flat, his voice emotionless.

'Who said I was having an affair?'

Does that mean he is?

I take a deep breath. I will sound unhinged.

'A website called Influenza. Someone on there said you'd been "handsy" with an intern.'

I try to say this casually, as though my source is unquestionable.

His face turns angry and for a moment I don't even recognise him. He's a stranger in the street.

'A website? Like some Instamum gossip? Jesus, Lo. I can't do this right now.'

He gathers his key and wallet and walks away without looking at me. I hear him give Scout a kiss on the head and tell her he's off to buy some milk, leaving me standing there alone, both hands on my stomach.

'Mummy, I'm hungry,' says Scout.

'Just a minute.'

I breathe out, stir the pasta and return it to the hob, because one of us has to feed our daughter.

It's been two hours and he's still not back.

I fed Scout and bathed her and put her to bed and as she asked, 'When's Daddy coming home?' I felt like an abandoned housewife and pictured expensive lawyers and stern talks about visitation rights and him living in a flat with a twenty-two-year-old.

I've been on Influenza ever since. I'm at the kitchen table with just the glow of my laptop screen as the views edge up. It's still under 10,000 and has gone quiet. No comments for twenty minutes. I keep scrolling back to the bit about Johno. Only one user picked it up.

turd_is_the_word says: What? In the bogs with an intern? It's like slut Cluedo!

Blahblahblah says: Ha!

turd_is_the_word says: Ohmigod, do you think she knows? Maybe he's allowed!?!? 🕵️

Blahblahblah says: It wouldn't surprise me.

Offices are perfect for affairs: everyone dressing their best and expected to be charming and pleasant. Those things don't happen at home among the debris of raising a child and losing yourselves in grief.

I hear his key in the lock. He drags his feet over the mat. Was he really upset, or was he fixing up his story?

He comes to the kitchen.

'Hi. Can I put the light on?'

'I don't mind.'

His voice is low now. Quiet. I can't read the emotion in it. He comes over and sits opposite me, like this is a negotiation.

'Lo, I haven't even got an intern.'

'What about Eilis?'

'Eilis?'

'The new girl. Whose clothes don't fit?'

'She's a finance assistant.'

'Her job title doesn't really matter to me, Johno.'

He lets out an exasperated little half-smile and I get a faint scent of beer and mints.

'Lo, can you please just explain to me where this has come from?'

I highlight the relevant bits and turn around my laptop. He leans over, reads and then he looks at me.

'Is that it?'

I just stare at him. I stare at him and I don't know. I want to be certain that it's lies or be certain that it's true.

'Lo, I mean . . .'

He makes a few, quiet gasping noises like the words won't form.

'. . . Who even is Blahblahblah anyway?'

'I don't know, but she knows a lot about you.'

'No, she doesn't, Lo.'

His voice is stern now. Maybe I'm pushing too far, but I've broken through something and there's no turning back. He sits down and raises his hands above the keyboard.

'Can I just see who she is?'

I give a shallow nod and he clicks around, finding other threads she's commented on.

'She's said here that someone called @SuperStarMum[La!] has had botox. Is that true?'

'I don't know.'

He clicks around a little more.

'Here, she says her good friend saw Davina McCall shoplifting from a newsagent's. Is that true?'

'I don't know.'

'Well, neither do I. But does it seem likely, do you think? Would Davina McCall need to shoplift?'

'Probably not.'

He pulls a slightly exaggerated grin and opens the palm of his hands. I feel a haze shift in my head. But I also feel a little stupid.

'You could've just been looking up her history, in the pub, on your phone.'

'Yes, I could. Would you like to check my browser history?'

He takes out his phone and slides it over and I look away. Why do I think the worst of the man I used to think the best of?

'Lo, look, I know the work thing is a shock, but do you really think I've been having an affair?'

Maybe. Probably not.

'No.'

He smiles and shrugs. He's waiting for me to apologise.

'It's just that there are some things on there they do know.'

'Like what?'

'Like how much I'm getting paid.'

I scroll back to show him.

'Are those numbers accurate?'

'Near enough.'

'Wow. If I'd known that I'd have quit months ago.' He smiles sheepishly.

I don't smile back.

'But it means they know me. They're people who know me.'

'Maybe. Or they're in the industry and guessing. Or they overheard some gossip in a pub. But what does it matter?'

'It's just not nice when it's about you.'

'I know, Lo, but really, what harm can it do?'

27

DECEMBER

DYLAN

It's damp and misty as I walk through Soho to meet Cal, one of those days that feel like you're out at sea.

I spent twenty minutes trying to work out what to wear this morning, before deciding that my book about an abused woman with no money sounds best coming from an abused woman with no money, so I've come as one of those. I am being my true self.

The pavement is still wet from heavy rain earlier, and I can feel a little bit of dampness in my right plimsoll. I went with these shoes partly because they feel simple and writerly, but mostly because I don't have any others.

Maybe I should call him Callum, actually, not Cal. They call him Callum under the blurry little headshot on the website.

But I'm having a meeting with a publisher in Soho, and that might be the best thing I've ever said in my entire life.

I think this might be the first meeting I've ever had that won't just be someone asking me if I can serve tea or operate a phone, and I want to tell everyone I've ever known, in case this is as good as it gets.

Right now it's a thing that's happening: I'm having a meeting with a publisher called Callum. That sounds good and exciting and, 'oh jeez, Dyl, aren't you a bit more interesting than you look.'

But in an hour that'll be gone. Then it might be, 'I had a meeting but it didn't work out,' which is probably what anyone would expect. Maybe it's what I expect.

I walk past Liberty, with all its old timber bits on the walls, like the place is either 400 years old and Shakespeare shopped there, or it was made to look that way, like they do with footballers' houses in Essex.

Then down Carnaby Street, and onto the cobbles of Broadwick. It's like a holiday now, being in town, because my whole life is within a fifteen-minute walk of our front door: school, park, supermarket, home-work-bed. The little circuit of me.

So I stop for a minute, breathe it all in. I am having a meeting with a publisher in Soho and it hasn't gone wrong yet.

What I really want to do is tell Lo, but it's been a bit hard to tell her anything recently. She's been flitting in and out the gates, dragging Scout behind her, off to do work things or with her face in her phone, no time for playdates, hasn't answered my message about the Etisk post. We can't have chatted for more than ten minutes since the night at hers, and now it's barely a nod as she flaps past. It's like we work together and copped off at the Christmas party but she'd rather forget about it.

I only ever see Johno in the park now if Scout's out to play, and he spends most of the time on his phone, pacing about the place saying, 'How about I follow up next week,' like he's suddenly flogging double glazing.

It shouldn't matter to me that Lo knows about today, but this might be one thing I have that she doesn't, and I can't just message her 'Hello, I'm having a meeting with a publisher in Soho, darling,' because that would make me a gloaty twat.

But I do want to say hello, so I tap out a text message. *'Hey, Lo. All OK?'*

I always wait after I message her, like something will come straight back, but it never does. So I walk on for my meeting in Soho with a publisher called Callum, saying it over and over in my head.

The place he chose is called 'Baguetterie', and on the website it says they only do baguettes and soft drinks and that's it. Ham baguette, cheese baguette, mixed baguette and nothing else. A 'holler back to the dignified simplicity of the *paysan*,' it says, but with baguettes that cost seven quid.

I get to the place and I'm two minutes early, so I spin Insta for a little flood of feelings.

@Jacar&aring

Thank GOD someone is speaking about real life.

@Inthem-o-o-o-ment

Oh @one__day__soon, I don't know who you are but I think I love you.

And one from my keenest follower.

@hopingwaiting247

I just want you to know that you're an inspiration. Your words really lift me up. Bit surprised you're friends with @the__lo__down__ to be honest.

Why, what's wrong with Lo?

'DYLAN!'

A man is stood next to me, leaning forward, smiling. He's got on a long scarf and a big beige mac and looks like he's auditioning for *Dr Who*.

'Hi,' I say.

He throws his head back, grins, stands his full height, and that must be 6'4', with a face that dances as he speaks. He looks older than his photo, maybe early fifties.

'SUCH a relief. I've got a terrible habit of introducing myself to the wrong people.' He starts each sentence with a shout, like he's snapping his fingers for attention.

'Callum?'

'YES! So good to meet you.'

He's slim, sounds a bit posh. He leans forward, puts his arm on my shoulder, kisses my cheek, and I step back, but he doesn't seem to notice. He smells expensive, of oak and spice.

'I thought it must be you, standing all alone.'

'Yes, hello, it's me.'

I smile at him, stand awkwardly.

'Shall we bag a baguette? On us?'

'Let's!'

He opens the door, steps aside, waving me in with a smile and a nod. The place has little circular, red, brass-ringed tables like they do in pictures of Paris and the staff all have white shirts and black waistcoats, but it's basically just a sandwich bar. We walk up to the counter and he orders straight away.

'Ham baguette and a double espresso for me, please.'

He looks my way.

'What do you fancy? Pretty limited selection, but that's the charm.'

'Mixed baguette and a cappuccino please.'

I never drink coffee, but it feels more writerly than tea. We stand in silence for a bit, Callum staring forward. Then he turns to me, like he's forgotten something important.

'And how was your journey in?'

'Fine, just got the Tube. You?'

'Yes, train in, Tube down, nip about town, then homeward.'

We stand there for a bit, and I wonder what to say. I feel like I should have something: a joke or an observation. Something to fix in his head that I am writerly.

But I have nothing to say about trains or Norwich, so I just stare at my feet, then at the counter and then up at him, my eyes running this little route like I am thinking deep, writerly thoughts when really I'm just praying for the food to arrive and hoping my cheeks don't go red.

I feel a little prickle run up my neck as he stands there, then he crosses one foot over in front of the other, leans his hand on the counter, smiles at me and I smile back.

Should I say it's cold out?

No. He knows it's cold out, that's why he's wearing a coat.

Maybe it was warmer in Norwich.

But Norwich is not the Med, it is just Norwich.

I start to open my mouth, but there's nothing there, so I close it again.

The food and coffees are placed on the counter and Callum leads the way to one of the tiny round tables. He sits, sighs, smiles at me. He is already fascinating, odd; this man who might change my life.

'I am SO GLAD you sent us *The Women Who Watch On*.'

'Well, thanks, I'm glad you like it.'

'Oh, I do. Truly, I do.'

It feels strange, hearing someone else say the name of it. I don't think I've ever heard that before, but just hearing it come from someone else's mouth makes it more solid; no longer my scribbles. Not my little vanity exercise or a therapeutic fantasy, but a real thing that others might read. A thing I might see in a shop and turn to Noah and say, 'Look, it's Mummy's book.'

Callum smiles again, stares, and there's a silence. He takes a bite of his baguette, savours it, and the quietness lingers, so I ask him:

'What did you like the most?'

He nods, chews a bit and his face dances all over the shop as though this is an excellent question, and he can't wait to answer, but he just happens to have food in his mouth, and now I wish I hadn't asked because it makes me look thoughtless. He chomps, swallows.

'I was so taken with Elaine's resistance. Her perseverance. And also, of course, there's a nice, gory murder at the end.'

He smiles. No one has ever spoken to me like this before and I don't know what to say. My eyes look down, I feel ridiculous, like this is a joke. Like there's a hidden camera somewhere and an audience pissing themselves with laughter.

'Really, Dylan, I liked it a lot.'

'Thanks.'

'How much of it is true?'

'Well, it's a story.'

'But based on your experiences?'

'A bit. I've never stabbed anyone.' I smile at him.

'Well, that IS good news.' He smiles back.

'But I have thought about it.'

His smile goes and he doesn't say anything, and I think I sound mad. I was trying to be all coy and intriguing, but now he thinks I sit alone at home, dreaming up ways to stab people.

'But the life she has,' I say, 'I know that. Some of it.'

He nods.

'And what's your situation?'

'Well, I'm a single mum with an abusive ex.'

His eyes narrow, he nods his head, does his best to look sympathetic, so I continue.

'Not really violent,' I say. 'But controlling. And also a bit violent. Sometimes. Or just rough, really. No cuts and bruises, just . . .'

And I don't know why I'm telling him this. He doesn't need to know, Dyl.

'I understand, I think. And is he still around, lurking somewhere?'

'I don't know.'

'Would it put you in danger being out there, if we did publicity?'

He looks concerned, stares straight at me.

'I could use a pen name? Stay out of sight.'

Callum looks at me a little longer.

'Be anonymous?'

'Yes.'

'Maybe.'

He says it slowly, like it's a puzzle he needs to think about. It feels like some kind of therapy session and I'm not sure what I expected. I just want him to publish my book. Give me a deal and make me an author, Callum!

He smiles a little, changes the subject, and does his little shout to move the conversation on.

'AND TELL ME, where did you grow up?'

'South of London. In the "burbs".'

'Just like Elaine.' He smiles, continues. 'I was really taken with the struggle of her early life.'

'Yes.'

'Was much of that from personal experience?'

I'm not sure what he wants, why he's asking. He looks at me a little longer.

'A bit.'

He nods again.

248

'That authenticity really comes across.'

I nod and smile back, but it feels like he wants more, so I give it to him.

'My dad also killed himself, and I left home at seventeen, too.'

His face turns down, saddened, like I'm injecting my tragedy into someone else again.

'That must've been very hard,' he says. 'I can't imagine what you and your mother must've gone through.'

'Yes. More for me than her, I think. She moved on pretty quickly. But we all grieve in different ways.'

He looks at me, doesn't know what to say, and I don't know if this is exactly the sort of thing he wants to hear, or if he thinks I'm an idiot. After a moment, he picks up his baguette and has another bite.

'How's your baguette?' he says, mid-chew.

'Great.'

I take a bite to prove it and we both chew silently until he swallows and raises a finger as though something has just occurred to him.

'Also, we've been very impressed with your social-media presence. That is a fast-growing audience you have there.'

'Thanks.'

'Really shows there's an appetite for these under-told tales of austerity life.'

'Yes.'

'Will you continue to post?'

'Definitely.'

'Oh, that's good. And you don't have an agent yet?'

'No.'

'Well, maybe best. Our budgets are very small, so why give some to a stranger, eh?'

'Yes.'

I smile at him, try not to speak for a moment.

'WELL, Dylan,' he sits upright, 'I think we WOULD like to publish your book. There's some work needed, but I think it is a vital and authentic tale of the kind too rarely told. The world needs more of these voices, and I'd like you to be ours. Will you let us publish it?'

A rush of warmth runs from my belly to my head, and I practically hop in my seat.

'Ooh, umm, lemme think . . .'

I do a little act, pretending for a moment that this isn't the most wonderful sentence I've ever heard, but he looks shocked and I don't think he gets it, so I blurt it out, 'Yes, of course!'

It comes out squeally. Like I'm a schoolgirl being given a pony. But I am wanted and I don't remember the last time I felt that from anyone who wasn't Noah.

'Well, that is excellent news. Congratulations to us both!'

'Yes.'

I breathe out, feel my skin cool and realise how hot I had been.

'And what's the advance?'

'Well, there is one, so that's good.'

He laughs, goes silent.

'And how much is it?'

'Five thousand pounds?'

He says this as a question and I stare at him, fix my face, but my head is spinning. I don't know what I expected. I would do this for nothing, just to have the chance for people to read my work. But if I can flog water to people who already have taps, I can sell my book to him.

'That's quite low, according to my research.'

'Oh, well, the internet can be a bit misleading. It tends to take one tiny corner of the picture and pretend it is everything. People get very excited about big deals, but they are a tiny fraction of the—'

'Of course. But you like it?'

'Yes. Very much.'

'And it's an "under-told" tale.'

'Absolutely.'

'Then perhaps an advance closer to what you might pay someone who wasn't a single mum?'

'Ha! Well . . .'

Callum's face becomes serious.

'I have been authorised to go to ten thousand pounds.'

I smile, offer my hand, and he offers his. I shake it a bit too hard, wobbling the table. I feel a warm sting of something in my eyes. I just earned another five grand in twenty seconds. A laugh jumps out of me.

For the first time in my life I am someone and it feels good.

I say goodbye and we peck cheeks, and as I walk to the Tube, I can barely feel my limbs. It's like I'm floating along the soggy pavement. Clouds lie over London like a manky blanket, but I feel so light I might float off and I want to tell everyone around me. All these people walking past, all these strangers on the wet street, charging about on their way to meetings or shopping or dates. Right now, in this moment, just for once, my life is better than theirs.

Something amazing and good has happened to me that hasn't happened to them and I want to shout it, or dance, or sing in the middle of the street. I want to grab a stranger by the arm and say, 'Hello, I am the author Dylan Rayne.'

Or not Dylan Rayne. Something made up. But I am an author. I step into a doorway and watch the people flow past and I lean my whole body back, put my hand on the beige brick wall to run my palms over every lump and bump of the brickwork, feel the grit and sand in the cement.

Maybe I can be some crazy old dear who wears big dresses and writes all day?

Maybe I can be very earnest and always frown in interviews?

Maybe I should start wearing glasses?

'My first novel? Yes, such a long time ago. So heartening to hear all the tales from women who felt uplifted, given strength, able to finally leave those men.'

I watch the street and everyone trudging along, and I want to know what Noah is doing right now. I hope he is writing words. I hope he has his tiny little fingers around a thick pencil and is slowly, wonkily marking out his name. I want to wrap my arms around him and squeeze him until he wriggles and cackles and says, 'Mummy, stop!'

I want to be in the room with him, like some tiny, invisible spirit on his shoulder, whispering in his ear that anything is possible.

I am publishing a book, Noah, and you can be proud of me like I am of you, because it is not supposed to be a thing that happens to women like me and I made it real.

I breathe out, sigh a happy sigh, and there's a madness in my blood, little prickles that make me warm, not scared. I should buy him a treat tonight.

I step forward, start walking back to the Tube and join all the people plodding along, but I am different to them, just for now. I'm a firefly and they're all bluebottles. I will buy Noah ice cream tonight and cover it in chocolate sauce. I will get it from somewhere nice, not the corner shop.

I will walk through Soho after my meeting with my publisher Callum and find nice ice cream for my son.

I stroll along, trying to control myself, trying not to go mad but smiling anyway.

Get a grip now, Dyl, lots can still go wrong. I don't know what, but I'm sure it can.

And then I stop dead in the middle of the street.

I see myself reflected in the plate-glass window of a bookshop. Inside, there's a green blanket over little shelves with books all propped up, tinsel draped about, little cardboard Christmas trees and a few plastic elves flogging the festive bestsellers.

I step closer, look at my reflection, my lined skin and limp two-tone hair. I am tired and I am scrappy, but I am here. I am here and I have made it this far and that is a miracle.

My dad is dead and my mum is almost lost to me, and JD could be anywhere, but I am here and that is a miracle.

And soon, maybe, my book might be in there, with all those others, and I want to tell everyone.

So I take out my phone, step back as people swerve around me, and take a picture of the shopfront, my silhouette barely visible in the window. I flick to Instagram, and add a little caption for 9,210 people.

Exciting news. Can't say much, but one day soon it might be my work in there.

I hit upload, spin and wait.

No likes.

I spin again, three little red hearts, spin again, seven more splotches of digital love and a comment.

@hopingwaiting247
Ohmigod! You've got a book deal? Already! SO DESERVED. I can't wait to read it.

I laugh. Maybe it is deserved.

I spin again, three more hearts. That's twenty-two in two minutes and a post of mine has never gone so well.

And it's silly, but I hope Lo sees it.

I just feel like maybe she'd be proud.

And might finally realise that I'm worth more than she thought.

28
LO

The local café feels like a sauna this afternoon. Condensation
creeps down the window and to the left of us sits a man with a
moustache teased like Salvador Dali's. There's gold tinsel deck-
ing the pop-art prints on the walls.

Scout is eating a croissant, the crumbs tumbling down her
school uniform and onto the floor. Every time someone walks
in, they shake their coat and droplets of rain splatter onto our
table. We are here as a treat, but she is weary.

I give her my wallet. She used to take all the cards and receipts out and reinsert them, one by one, but now she prefers
to pretend it's a mobile phone, tapping at imaginary buttons.
Today she slumps in her chair and hands the wallet back.

'I'm bored,' she says.

'I've just got to do some work, Scout, and then I'll be with
you, OK?'

I say 'just' a lot. I just need a minute, I just need a second.
And when she says, 'Has it been a minute yet?' I lie to her and
say no.

'OK,' she says sullenly. 'Can I have a treat?'

She knows I won't refuse. I get up to buy her a Caramel bar

and she urgently unwraps the gold and orange foil as I swipe to WhatsApp.

Another message from Dyl, unanswered messages from Amara, Mum, Johno. When I try to reply to people, my head freezes and my thumbs can't move. I say so much to strangers that I don't know what to say to friends. I just wish they'd leave me alone for a minute. It feels like there's always someone needing something from me.

I'll see Dyl in the playground soon enough. Johno's done most of the school runs, enjoying his new 'work/life balance'. He has taken a hot desk in a place with exposed pipes and free coffee that he calls 'HQ'.

I have five messages from Jenn asking for confirmation that I'm still posting the WeAreFemForm ad at 5.00 p.m. Her most recent is in capitals: *'LO, YOU THERE?'* with a meme of Forrest Gump running and a row of smiley faces gurning through the cracked screen. It's her job to make sure I post on time. I just wished she'd been as thorough briefing me about it.

In a draft post, I have the WeAreFemForm video and the agreed caption.

I feel so hugely privileged to be part of this campaign. It's not often you come across a brand that's willing to go beyond selling, and WeAreFemForm is one of those. Having experienced period poverty for one cycle, I truly get it and it's a heartbreaking reality for so many – too many – young women living without basic sanitary products. It's bloody embarrassing, it's bloody humiliating. It's got to bloody stop, and for every pack sold, WeAreFemForm will donate 5% of their profits to charity. Here's to changing the future for all our girls. Don't be one of the women who watch on ☉.
#periodofchange #periodpoverty #WeAreFemForm #ad

Hard to believe that 100 words could take eight rounds of amends and edits. I got less feedback on my uni dissertation.

Uploading feels as routine as sending an email, not broadcasting to 112,000 people. I got thousands more follows after Influenza kicked off, but I don't know who is out there anymore.

I felt like I used to, at the beginning. It felt like a community of women hacked off with a working world that shafts mothers, but now it feels like standing on a rigged stage and speaking into a dark abyss. The bigger your audience gets, the less human you become, and it's impossible to be personal to 112,000 people.

But more followers means Jenn can charge higher fees, so maybe I don't have to do it for so long. Three to five years, perhaps. Make a big dent in that mortgage, then put Instagram down and cuddle my daughter. Or her and a sibling.

I rub my belly, hit post and put the phone in my bag like it's a smoking gun. I sit there teasing my hair, seeing what comes free.

Scout has ripped the biscuit wrapper into small pieces and is throwing them onto the floor. There's a carpet of pastry crumbs and foil beneath our table and I sigh louder than necessary, kneeling down to sweep it all up with a serviette. There are two mums to my right whispering to each other as their babies gnaw rice cakes. I wonder if they know what's being said. I wonder if they're commenting.

Scout huffs and I look at her chocolate-covered mouth. I wipe it with a clean serviette as she does an exaggerated frown.

'What did you do today?'

She looks at me like I've asked her to recite the Ten Commandments in Greek.

'Did you have a good day?'

'Yeah.'

She stares down and continues to throw small balls of foil onto the floor. One of the mums on the next table watches on.

'Scout, can you stop that please, it's making a mess,' I say, loud enough for the other mothers to hear.

I take the biscuit wrapper off Scout and scrunch it into my empty coffee mug. She doesn't look up and slumps a little further in her chair and looks away from me. She has a sticker on her lapel that has a beaming squirrel holding a 'well done' sign and I try my nice voice.

'What did you get that sticker for?'

She slides deeper into her chair, the overhead lights accentuating the dark circles under her eyes, and ignores me. School is tiring for a four-year-old. I justify her surliness with exhaustion, in the way that all parents seem to when their children act out – 'He's just a little hungry' or 'She just needs an early night.' We wave off their behaviour in the way we never do for adults.

'Shall we head home?'

'OK,' she says meekly.

I slip my hand in hers, squeezing gently, and we both stand. She squeezes back and in an instant we are as connected as we once were in the womb.

The rain has stopped and we make our way into the sinking darkness of the afternoon.

'Can we go to Noah's house?'

'Not today, Scout.'

'But we've never been there and he hasn't been to our house for ages.'

'I know, but I've been working.'

We walk in silence for a minute and then Scout pulls my hand a little harder.

'Why are you always working?'

Her voice is accusatory, but also pleading.

'I'm not, Scout. I'm here now, aren't I?'

'But you're always on your phone. It doesn't count if you're on your phone.'

It's a little kick to the chest, a break in my breathing. A reminder that I haven't always 'got this', despite all the motivational quotes.

'It's not perfect, Scout, but I am here. Lots of mummies and daddies have other people picking their kids up, so you are very lucky, really.'

It feels like I'm mostly speaking to myself. She doesn't answer and we walk in silence, my mind flicking to the post because I need to check how it's going.

The darkness creeps around us so it already feels like night. There's a rubbish bag on the pavement that's been ravaged by a fox or a rat. Scout and I step over chewed packaging for some microwaveable dish and I get my phone out to check the time. It's 5.15 p.m. Johno should be home soon.

I flick to Instagram and a flood of red pours onto my screen. The post only has 156 likes but seventy-three comments. I feel my heart jump and I stop under an elm tree. Scout huddles into my thigh.

@Motherofhaggins

You can't be serious? Pretending to be poor to make money? This is the most tone-deaf thing I've seen here. It's embarrassing.

@Laura-Bafour-her-4

Lo, love everything you do but there is so much wrong with this.

@Roo{and}thebear!

How Lo can you go, eh? Cashing in on period poverty? Glaring middle-class privilege at its finest.

259

@Mum*Beam*

Who thought this was OK? Do better, Lois.

@Suze"79"

Hey, @Roo{and}thebear!, there's a real human here, everyone makes mistakes.

@spite-up-your-life

Thick as shit. Shame on WeAreFemForm, shame on you.

I feel a clench in my stomach. Like our plane has hit turbulence and dropped fifty metres. The back of my throat runs hot like I'm going to be sick. I can't get upset, I can't let the baby feel this.

'Mummy, I'm cold,' says Scout, tugging my hand. 'Can we go now?'

'Just wait!'

I snap at her and regret it. I squeeze her shoulder and hold my phone, the gentle buzz of activity continuing to heat my palm.

We walk, holding hands, down a small alley that has a graffitied heart on one side as I try to suck in air. I need to speak to Jenn. I go to text, but then press 'call'. It rings twice before she picks up and greets me with the gusto of a cheerleader.

'Hi, how are you doing?'

'Have you seen the post?'

I stand still in the alleyway, holding Scout tightly.

'No, what's up?' There's hesitation in her voice. She always checks my ads.

'Mummy, can we go?' Scout pulls her hand out of mine and I hush her again.

'It's getting a lot of negativity. What should I say?'

'A bit of kickback is totally normal on big campaigns like this, don't worry, it's all going to be fine. I might be able to catch the client before she leaves the office. Give me a minute and I'll call you back.'

'OK, I'll wait to hear from you.'

'Don't worry, it's all going to be fine!'

I hang up and check the post again: 115 comments. One faceless avatar has tagged a period-poverty charity. I flick to Influenza and walk on, Scout beside me.

On Influenza, there's a new thread called: 'How Lo can she go?' It started two minutes after my post.

I click through and there's a GIF of my face on a bloody tampon and a speech bubble shouting, 'Bloody good show!' I scroll through as my body guides me home. I bump into a man in a big puffa jacket who tuts as he takes out one of his ear pods and carries on. I hold onto Scout's limp hand and walk while looking down at the glow of the phone in the misty evening light.

Floggetyflog says: What the hell has she just done? It feels like Christmas came early. Get yourselves to Insta and let her know.

Barefaced says: I'm a fan of Lo (ducks for cover) but I literally can't believe she pretended to be poor for cash.

Slashintheattic says: My daughter is at the same school as Scout and I'm what you'd call 'poor' in her eyes. I smiled at her a few weeks ago and she looked right through me.

We reach the gate of our house.

'Scout, I'm so sorry.'

There's silence.

'Mummy's just got something important to do at work. But I shouldn't have shouted at you. I shouldn't have been cross.'

She doesn't say anything and I kneel down to hug her limp

little body, absorbing her warmth. It starts to rain again as I turn the key.

'Did you get milk?' Johno says in greeting. He's on his laptop in the kitchen.

'No,' I say.

'Oh. I messaged.'

He scrapes the chair against the crumb-flecked floor tiles, walks over and pecks me on the cheek, ruffles Scout's hair, grabs his coat.

'I'll go now,' he says.

I want him to stay and hold me. I want him to gently squeeze the worry out of me. I want to tell him I feel like I'm naked on a floodlit football pitch, with darkness closing in. I want to tell him they're right: I'm thick, I'm money-grabbing, I'm an embarrassment and there's probably a sick fuck wanking to a photo of Scout. I want to tell him I need to know what they're saying, because they are right. They're the only ones telling me the truth.

But Scout is here, so I let him go.

As he's leaving, he calls over his shoulder:

'There's pasta bake in the oven, if you want to get Scout started, and we can eat later?'

Then he closes the door loudly behind him.

'Mummy, what's faster, dust or fire?'

Scout is at the dining table now, playing with Blu-Tack.

I refresh the Influenza thread and there are thirty-four more comments. I flick to Instagram and there are fifty-eight. Jenn is typing on WhatsApp.

'MUMMY, what's faster, dust or fire?'

Scout is waving her hands and has made herself cross-eyed.

'I don't know, Scout.'

I don't have an answer for her. She looks dejected and starts moulding small pieces of Blu-Tack into people, lining them up like soldiers. Her own little faceless army.

I open a cupboard and Tupperware falls out, clattering to the floor. I breathe in and carefully restack everything. My mind feels like it's on an outpost with weak phone signal.

Two missed calls from Amara and a text.

'Just seen your post. Happy to sense-check anything. Love you. Always here. Xxx'

I need to take it down.

Johno crashes through the door.

'I got a bottle of red.'

He waves the wine like it's a regional football trophy. He's been gone for fifteen minutes and I haven't moved, just had my face to my phone. He scans the scene, picking up the lack of progress.

'It's been a rubbish day,' I say.

'What happened?'

He looks worried, like I'm bleeding or bruised. I've never seen him look at me that way. What can he see in me?

I catch a reflection of myself in the kitchen window and my skin is sallow, my eyes blank.

'I'll tell you later. Let's just get her to sleep.'

'Why don't you take some time upstairs, and I'll get Scout down?'

'NO, I want Mummy.'

Scout runs over and clings to my leg. I want to shake her off like she's a muddy puppy and guilt floods over me for thinking these thoughts. I'm still holding my phone and scoop her up, trying to squeeze the last few hours of casual neglect out of her memories. She squeezes me around the neck with all her might.

'Scout, Scout. Mummy can't breathe.'

'I love you, Mummy.'

Johno goes to dish up dinner, and over Scout's shoulder I refresh the magenta screen.

There's a screen grab of a *Mail Online* article with my face on it.

Scout invents a song, which she repeats in my ear:

'Mummy rhymes with tummy, Mummy rhymes with tummy.'

The headline reads 'How Lo can you go? Followers FURIOUS with Instagram star "pretending to be poor" while being paid 12 GRAND'.

Tears press against the back of my eyes.

'Mummy, why are you crying?'

'I'm not.'

'Yes, you are.'

Scout is still in my arms and leans back, knocking the phone from my hand so it lands with a crack on the floor.

'Scout, stop it!'

It's a mad, desperate shout and I almost throw her down as I go to my phone. The screen has a hundred little spindles spiralling out from the centre, like someone has taken a bat to a shop window. I swipe and get flecks of cracked glass. I swipe again and there's a flicker, but it works. I swipe Instagram and it refreshes and for a second my muscles loosen.

I look up and Scout is dead still, staring at her shoes and weeping.

Johno looks at me like he's witnessed a car crash, holding Scout's dinner plate with a steaming portion of pasta bake.

29

DYLAN

Noah is asleep at the end of our perfect day. After seeing Callum, I literally ran into the playground, scooped him up and we skipped for about twelve paces until I felt too knackered and he felt too daft.

As we walked down the street, I showed him the little tub of chunky-fudge ice cream and I thought his head might explode. When I told him I was writing a book, he must've seen the happiness in my eyes, because he just wrapped himself around my leg. Or maybe that was for the ice cream.

Either way, as he sleeps, the air coming through his slightly parted little lips, for the first time I can see a future for us.

I just wish I could tell Lo, but it feels more and more like she's just put me in a little box, set aside now that she's had her fun.

I flick to my phone. More floods of red for my book post.

@Janet-from-the-block
Ooooh, what could it be! So exciting!
@Claire&thegang27
Congrats babe, whatever it is!?!?!

I didn't think anyone would care. If I'm honest, it felt a bit gloaty, a bit humblebrag. But people do care. They care about me.

I flick to the top of my feed and a video appears of Lo's face as I leave Noah and walk through to the kitchen to watch.

She's glorious, really.

She beams down the camera lens with that thick brown hair tumbling to her shoulders, those blue eyes sparkling. She's in the same outfit as the day we had our drinks and under those lights her make-up is perfect. Her cheekbones look sculpted, her lips all full, like she's an old-fashioned movie star.

She's in profile, talking to someone off camera:

'I've experienced period poverty . . .'

That's weird. I mean, when?

They cut to other women, dipping their hands in red paint, some saying the same line, some sticking handprints on a white wall. It's a bit odd, the whole thing. And then finally I see her again, staring straight into the camera.

'There's no shame in struggling, there's shame in ignoring. Don't be one of the women who watch on.'

What?

I roll my thumb back, replay what I've just seen.

'. . . the women who watch on.'

I stare for a second, and it's like I'm seeing things.

'. . . the women who watch on . . .'

Those are my words, Lo.

I feel warmth in my throat, emptiness in my belly.

'. . . the women who watch on . . .'

I put my phone down on the counter because my hand is shaking and I watch it again.

'. . . the women who watch on . . .'

I don't understand. It's like she's reached into me and pulled something out.

I wrote that book by hand.

On crappy little notepads and in different coloured pens stashed under the mattress to hide it from JD.

I wrote it when he was out drinking and had locked the flat from the outside.

I wrote it when he'd finished with me and had fallen asleep.

I wrote it for two years, and then I saved for a year more to buy a crappy laptop and type out every single word.

Those are my words, Lo.

They might be the only thing that is truly mine.

Not rented, not borrowed, not on tick. From my head and my life and you've taken them. What is wrong with you?

I watch it again, and I don't know what to do.

Is this plagiarism? How did she even know? Did I tell her the name of the book?

Maybe it doesn't matter. Maybe I'm being stupid.

But I stare at her, saying my words over and over again, and every time, I feel a little burn in the back of my throat.

I pick up my phone and call her, but she doesn't reply. Her phone is like an extra limb to her, so she's seen the call. She's watching my name pop up right now, looking at it and thinking, 'Nope, not talking to you.'

Jesus Christ, Lo.

Is that it? I've served my purpose? A few playdates for your kid, rent my son's cut-price face, rob my words and it's time to move along, Dyl.

I need to know if I'm going mad.

I flick to Instagram, flick to my messages, and right at the top sits @hopingwaiting247. She's anonymous too, no posts and only a few followers.

I send her a DM.

'Hey. Can I ask you something?'

I send it and wait and she answers straight back, like she must have been scrolling right at that minute.

'Ohmigod, hi! Of course you can! I think you're great! (Oops, fangirl, sorry!)'

@one__day__soon 'Why did you say you were surprised I was friends with Lo Knox?'

@hopingwaiting247 'Well, I dunno, I mean, it's just like she is so much the opposite of everything you are fighting for.'

The only things I'm fighting for are my boy, my book and some water-cooler sales, so I message her again.

'What do you mean?'

@hopingwaiting247 'Well, you are real and honest. No one's life is like hers, really, but all the women we see are just like her. No one talks about our lives and you're the only one doing that. Women like her, they say all this stuff about smashing the system, but they're just flogging us shit we don't need! (Sorry, it gets me a bit wound up ☹).'

I stare at her words, read them again. She's typing a new message.

@hopingwaiting247 'Why do you ask?'

@one__day__soon 'Have you seen Lo's WeAreFemForm ad?'

@hopingwaiting247 'YES! That's exactly what I mean. She thinks it's funny, acting poor, in an ad for thousands of pounds!'

@one__day__soon 'Well, the words she uses, "don't be one of The Women Who Watch On", she got that from me.'

@hopingwaiting247 'I SAW! From one of your early posts, about *being too skint for frozen peas! I nearly cried when I read that first time. I thought it was weird she said it.'*

So that's where. Lo lifted it straight from my post. She is shameless.

@one__day__soon *'I just wonder: is it that bad, what she's done?'*
@hopingwaiting247 *'Oh my God it's terrible! It's appropriation. All we've got is our words. It's who we are! I am SO sorry this has happened to you.'*

She types again.

@hopingwaiting247 *'Oh my God: is it the name of your book too? Is that why you wrote it capitals? If she's taken the name of your book that is horrible. Probably plagiarism.'*

She is a stranger and she can see how bad this is. My friend used my boy in her ad for a fraction of his worth and now she's used my words. Stolen them. Earned money from them.

@one__day__soon *'Thanks. I just wondered if I was being unreasonable.'*
@hopingwaiting247 *'No way! She stole your words! She owes you. You are NOT being unreasonable.'*

I put my phone down.

I was such an idiot to think I could have something that was mine.

My jaw clenches as I think of her, coiled on that green velvet sofa. She didn't need to take this. She has so much, and I had this one thing.

I dial her number again and no reply.

Well, you can ignore my calls, Lo, but you can't avoid the school gates forever.

The caretaker works his key in the lock and Noah runs ahead to line up as I follow behind to wait by his side. I watch the playground fill, seeing what lies around me, watching for Lo because she needs to put this right.

The space begins to surge with bodies. Kids line up behind Noah, some saying hello, some not. Some have a parent by their side but a few get left by grown-ups quick to turn around and run off to work.

I can't see Scout yet, or Lo or Johno. Ms Carole arrives for Noah's class, but still I can't see Lo. The playground is heaving now, perhaps a thousand people. Bodies keep crossing over my vision and still I can't see her.

'Right, children, in we go,' says Ms Carole.

'Bye, bye, Mummy,' says Noah.

I dart down to give him a kiss on the top of his head.

'Bye, Noh, have a great day.'

Is she hiding from me? The kids troop past and there's Scout, chatting to another little girl, but no Lo and no Johno, either.

I look through the playground but can't see her anywhere, so I jog towards the gate. Maybe I can catch her on the way out.

There are bodies in the way, and I'm trying to hop around them, keeping an eye out for her. A dad walks right in front of me and I have to break my stride not to bang into him. There's a mum with a double buggy and I have to skip around her.

I get to the gate and I watch them all traipse out, but she's nowhere.

Jesus, Lo.

Are you actually hiding from me now?

30

LO

We enter the school gates in a rush because we're late and I pull the hood up on my khaki duffel coat because eyes are on me.

Or maybe they aren't.

Maybe no one cares about my odd corners of the internet, but I feel watched. Is the woman I ignored here? Is she watching now, wondering if I've read the threads?

Scout's hand slips out of mine as she joins her line, and I don't get a chance to kiss her goodbye as she runs off into another world that doesn't involve me.

Then I turn away and head into mine. I pull out my phone and sink my neck and chin into my duffel coat and turn my eyes down. We all flow out, parents off to their other lives, me with my hood up like a fugitive.

Last night, Johno told me to just delete the app. Just stop checking the threads. But deleting the app doesn't remove my footprint. Deleting the app doesn't delete my mistakes. Ignoring the threads doesn't delete the shame. It just deletes my voice.

I look up to cross the road and the lollipop lady gives me a smile. She is round and grey and has been doing this job for thirty years. I nod and cross, wondering if she was a good mother. The sort to put pants and vests on the radiator to warm them, and make chocolate Rice Krispie cakes on rainy days.

I thank her and walk on to the park. I scan the tarmacked area and spot an empty bench. There's a discarded can of Strongbow next to me and a memorial plaque to a man called Cecil Bambridge that reads: 'Rest a while and smile'. I sit down and tumble into the familiar magenta-grey glow.

> **Higherchair says:** Have you seen @Bodyprotest! has just posted about her on Insta? It's brutal. Grab the popcorn, ladies.
>
> **Blissfullyaware says:** Good on her. BP is a real activist, whereas Lo is a saleswoman preying on the vulnerable. Popcorn grabbed, sitting tight, Lo is going down.

I flick back to Instagram and see my thickly made-up face on @Bodyprotest!'s feed. I look like a stranger, a caricature, a gruesome version of myself: like a slab of meat on the counter, lopped from all its limbs.

She says it's 'poverty porn . . . desperate appropriation . . . tone-deaf . . . what fun, earning twelve grand while pretending to have a poor vagina.'

She's right and I know she is.

Jenn's smiling face bursts through my phone screen and I press the red cross to push away her call. Strangers pass me, heads buried into coats and scarves. My heart pounds against my ribcage and I wonder if others can hear it because it's so loud. I want to message everyone and tell them that they're right: I'm stupid, I am selling my child on the internet.

I want to tell them they've won. I want the noise to stop, I can't hear myself think. I gulp for air and I want to press delete.

Darkness descends on my eyes like a dropping curtain. Flashes of light dart across my eyelids like sparklers against a night sky. I hold onto the cold, metal armrest on Cecil's bench, trying to breathe, but I can't get enough air in my lungs. I feel like I'm drowning in front of an audience: a faceless crowd stood on the pier, popcorn in hand, as water fills my lungs.

But it's not water, it's red paint.

A woman in a suit and a beige trench coat walks past and chucks a used coffee cup in the bin before staring back at her phone, and I wonder if she knows what they're saying.

I breathe deeply, but I can't get enough air in.

I just need to do something to make them stop. I need to show them that I'm not an @tag but a human. That I know this was a mistake, but I have friends who know me and what I've done for them.

I need to say something to make them go away, because my lungs are in a vice and they can't open enough to pull down the oxygen I need.

The vice is getting tighter and it will soon stop my heart, but my heart is enraged, rattling like a drum roll, and now I can't see. I can't see past patches of grey spots, misting over my eyes, and now my hands are shaking.

Shaking like it's freezing, like it's minus 20 and I'm naked in the snow.

31

DYLAN

I walk from the school gates, my face staring down at my phone, and I flick to her feed to see where she is, see what version of her life she is selling today, but there's nothing new.

So, for the first time in a while, I flick to Influenza.

And suddenly she is everywhere. There are thousands of comments, half a dozen threads. Stuff about Johno, about Scout. They're tearing her apart. They hate her and they're telling her, and each one is an anonymous, blank face.

They're saying she's a fake, and she makes mugs of vulnerable women. They're saying Johno touched up a girl at work, and I remember how he looked at me, that morning.

They're calling it child abuse, what she does, using Scout in ads.

What I've done, too.

It's horrible, the way they're going for her. But the more I read, the more I see what I should've know all along: that she will do anything to make money and she doesn't care about anyone else.

And they don't even know that she's stolen my words. Used me and tossed me away like old gum.

A man pushes past as I read and I instinctively want to hit him. I clench my fists, nails digging into my palms, and breathe in.

It is appalling that she would do this, be so calculating. To pretend to be so caring, while she casually fleeces me over Noah's picture, casually robs my words so she can earn a fortune off them in some horrible ad.

And all with that smile on her face.

She never cared about me. I was just another character in a play that revolves around her.

I go to her feed, spin to refresh, stare again, see what she has to say for herself, see her face, saying my words.

And as I land on her feed, it's like my whole body hollows out.

There I am.

My face next to hers.

Both of us grinning.

Sat at her table like the best of pals. Geotagged Haringey.

And the caption.

I came here to help women. To help myself, too, when I felt like no one was listening. And when you all started to listen, well, I felt something. I felt understood and less alone. I make mistakes, just like the rest. But I try to help women every day, because this space is not just for me. It's ours. I am here to elevate others. Others like my friend Dylan (@one__day__soon) – a single mother raising her son alone, navigating hardships that I wouldn't even dare to imagine and who now has a platform of her own. These are the voices I elevate. So follow her, support her, raise her voice. I won't always get it right here, but you have my word that I will never stop learning and unlearning.

I feel like I can't stand. Like my limbs are empty.

I am anonymous for a reason, Lo.

You have to let me stay anonymous, Lo.

If he sees this, Lo.

Lo, if he sees this . . .

My heart punches in my chest and the prickles run up my neck and for a second it feels like I haven't got enough blood inside me. I dial her number, wait for her cheery, idiotic voice, but she doesn't answer, so I text her, my fingers beginning to shake.

'Lo: take my picture down IMMEDIATELY. You cannot use it. You do not have permission. Take it down now. You have no idea what you've done.'

I call and no reply. I call again, but nothing. She is looking at my name right now and thinking: *nope, done with you.*

Jesus, Lo, answer me.

You've told 112,000 people where I live, Lo. That's a big city's worth of people, Lo. You've got Scout in her school uniform on your feed, Lo. Anyone who sees that post can work out Noah's school in five minutes. Any one of those 112,000 people. All the ones on Influenza. All those casual scrollers.

Why are you doing this to me, Lo?

What have I ever done to you?

Because I tell you what, I will not go back to him.

I will not go back to him, because he held all of me and I am not that woman anymore. He held the money and he held my phone account and he kept my friends away. He told me Jordi was stoned and that's how he fell, and he told me Mum didn't care and he told me my dad killed himself to escape me, and every minute that picture is up brings him closer, Lo. I will not go back and I will not let him see my boy.

And if he tries, I will stab him right in the heart.

*

I'm at the gate and looking all around as the caretaker opens up. He nods and smiles, but I stare right through him because my eyes are puffy little balls in skin as white as flour.

I have both hands deep in my jacket pocket, and in my right palm, fingers tight around the handle, is my best kitchen knife.

Because if JD comes for us, I will make sure he never does it again.

He wouldn't have got here yet, there isn't the time, but still I wait, prowl the concrete, watch the place slowly fill, and he is nowhere.

Maybe he doesn't need me anymore. Maybe he doesn't care. Maybe no one wants me.

Your own dad danced on the tracks to get away from you, Dilly.

Noah's class comes out and I march right up and take him away, with Ms Carole looking all flustered.

'If parents could wait, please . . .'

But she's just a noise as I walk home with Noah and have my left hand around his wrist and he drags behind me while I look all about, with my other hand on the knife tucked in my pocket. I have called that woman four times and messaged seven and she is ignoring me, because she has a foul little heart and there is not another living soul who matters to her.

'Mummy, slow down!'

We get home and I close the door and breathe in through my nose and out through my mouth and Noah looks scared.

'Mummy, why are you angry with me?'

He has a tear rolling down his face.

I have never seen him look like this. It's like he doesn't know me and he looks shrunken.

'I'm so sorry, darling.'

I have so much to be sorry for and he doesn't even know.

'I'm so sorry.'

I ease my fingers off the knife for the first time in half an hour and pull him close and hug him and I never want to make him feel that way again. It's like something is scraping at my head from the inside and my forehead feels hot because I'm hurting my son.

'I promise you, I'm not angry.'

'But your face is angry.'

'I promise I was just thinking about work. I love you so much.'

'But you made me drop my sticker.'

'What sticker?'

'Coming home, you were going so fast I dropped my sticker.'

He just doesn't know. He just doesn't know how things are, because he's four and he shouldn't have to.

'I'm sorry, darling. Maybe we can get another one.'

'But it's from school. Me and Scout and Farhaan and Kiyana got gold stickers because our projects were the best.'

'Oh, well done, Noh Noh!'

He looks at me and I smile a giant smile because I love his face so much and I just laugh out loud. I laugh and a few tears tumble out. I hold him because his skin is so perfect and soft and there is no love like this. There is no need as great. It's like he has magnets in his belly and they pull me towards him.

It's like I am his protective shell and him a little turtle. But I also need him, because without him I'll be empty and rot away on the ground.

So I feed him and I hold him, my tiny boy with so much he

could be. I give him a bath and wash his hair. I dress him in pyjamas and put him to bed and then I sit on the floor while he's in bed and stroke his forehead with my index finger and whisper, 'Sleepy time.' Over and over, like I did when he was a baby.

And when Noah is gently sleeping, I sit on his bedroom floor and pull my phone from my pocket and look at the woman who is doing this to us.

I look at her with a breast pump on her tit pretending to save the world. I look at her swinging Scout upside down in that beautiful living room. I look at her stealing my words and using my boy's face and then serving me up to harm.

This is the best life Noah's ever had, and this is the best place we've ever been, and she has put it in danger.

@hopingwaiting247 'Oh my God, Dylan (sorry, can I call you that, now?) I've just seen her post. I can't believe she is doing this to you. She's doxxed you! It is so terrible what is happening to you. Such an invasion, to take someone's words and use them like she is using you.'

And then I look at Influenza and it tells me that she is rotten. That she will steal and lie and manipulate. That she will sell everything: her husband, her home and her child, all the babies that didn't live and anyone who passes through her life.

There are thousands of comments.

She's laughing at poor people.

She's exploiting her daughter.

And then it's 1.00 a.m. and I know I cannot run anymore and I cannot hide.

We will not leave our life, because there's nowhere we can go and this is the best life we've ever had.

This tiny little flat, my joke telesales job, all of this is the best we've ever had it and we just need help.

I need an army of people watching over me, because I shouldn't have to do it alone any more.

I need people to see what she has done to us and I need them to protect us.

So I tell them who she really is.

32

LO

My eyes are closed but my mind is awake and I feel a scratch at my bare shoulder. Scout sways sleepily with her night-night cup. She looks ruffled, like a little chick that's fallen out of its nest.

'I'm thirsty.'

My phone reads 4.56 a.m. and I have hundreds of notifications. If I don't get Scout back to sleep, she'll be up for the day.

'OK. Go back to bed and I'll bring you milk.'

I get out of bed and my limbs crack like glow sticks. I guide her back to her bed, past Johno noisily sucking air, and I use my phone to guide me downstairs to the kitchen, keeping my eyes partly closed. The light catches a photo of us on our wedding day, our smiles like ghosts in the semi-darkness.

The chill from the fridge makes me shiver. It smells of sagging salad leaves and strong cheese. I pour milk into Scout's cup, heat it up in the microwave, lean against the cold marble counter and reach for my phone: I've been mentioned in 198 Instagram comments. Things were dying down, the noise was quietening.

The microwave pings and my heart jabs into my chest.

Dyl has tagged me in a post.

I want the facts to be laid down. Today I read a post by Lois Knox @the__lo__down__ for a paid period-poverty campaign with the line 'Don't be one of the women who watch on.' If you can ignore the tone-deafness of a middle-class woman pretending to be poor, that's my line. They're my words. I wrote them here in a post two months ago (swipe left for original post) and she took them right out of my mouth. She took my emotional and mental labour and she profited from it with no recompense for me. But then she did something far worse. She used my face. Showed me off as her 'poor mate', geotagged on her feed. Revealed me to the world and stole the anonymity I relied on to hide from an abusive former partner. Maybe led him to my front door. To my son. To us. I befriended her, despite my doubts, and she has used me. She has done violence to me. More violence than he ever could, because I trusted her and she gave me hope. But I cannot sit in silence anymore and neither should you. Please don't just be one of the women who watch on.

I read it again and I don't understand. I don't recognise the woman being spoken about. She's a parody, a pantomime villain, she's inhuman.

How can Dyl lie?

How can Dyl lie so deliberately?

I read thousands of things a day. How could I know where it came from? Words don't become yours just because you use them on Instagram, Dyl.

And how could I lead someone to you, when you told me he was dead?

For God's sake, Dylan, you told me he was dead!

She's lying, but it doesn't matter, because who am I? I'm the enemy. I am privilege. Everyone sees the evil cartoon, and no one sees who I am, because they do not care and this will be the end of me.

This is how the mob will get me.

I put my phone face down on the counter and I'm cold and tears begin to run down my face.

I clasp my cheeks, feel my skull. A noise comes out of me and I slump to the cold floor, holding my knees to my chest.

'Mummy.'

I sit up and breathe in hard. Silhouetted against the kitchen door is Scout, looking bedraggled and lost.

'Mummy, you didn't come.'

She's standing away from me, looking unsure.

'Scout, I'm sorry,' I say, wiping damp hair from my face, hoping the darkness hides me. 'Your milk's ready, I'll bring it up now.'

'Mummy, why were you making that noise?'

And I don't know what to say, so I tell her the truth.

'Sometimes mummies can be sad. That's OK; you know? It's nothing to be scared of.'

'Why are you sad?'

She's leaning on one foot and swaying. I pause and can't think. She stares at me.

'Because Mummy has been misunderstood, Scout. Do you know what misunderstood means? It means people see one thing when you are another.'

'What people?'

'Just someone from work.'

I hug her tightly, and see my tears spill onto the rabbits on her pyjamas. She hugs me back and I scoop her up, carry her upstairs and tuck her up in bed with the milk, hoping this won't be a memory that lasts.

Then I creep back down to pick up my phone, the glare stinging my eyes, and tap into another world.

The morning light filters in through the shutters, and Influenza is feasting on my ineptitude. I'm a deer absorbed by the pull of headlights, waiting for something to hit me. Willing something to hit me, leave me crumpled on the bonnet. To give me an out and make it stop. Because if I'm in hospital, I'm safe. They'll take my phone away, they'll tell me I'm unwell and I need help. If I'm in hospital, this can end and maybe they will leave me alone then.

On Influenza someone shares a tabloid feature; headline: 'Instamum Lo Knox leads abusive ex to her single-mum best friend.'

The truth is irrelevant and nuance is lost.

I'm a figment, a dartboard, a repository for other people's rage, and the noise won't stop until the witch is dead and justice has been served.

And it's my fault and I can't breathe.

I look up and try to blink the tiredness away. I need to see Dyl. I need her to stop the lies. I need to look her in the eye because she can't see me. If she could, she wouldn't have done this. Her post has 7,678 likes and I wonder where she is right now. If she's in her kitchen, getting Noah's breakfast ready, fuelled by the attention.

Upstairs, our alarm goes off and I hear Johno stirring. For days he's been saying, 'ignore it and it'll go away,' and I can't hear it anymore, because it doesn't just go away. So I say nothing and he doesn't ask, because he can't hear me tell him our only source of income is tearing me apart.

I need the toilet and creak upstairs and in the toilet my urine is the colour of golden syrup. I stand in front of the mirror and don't recognise the reflection. I don't yet look pregnant, just bloated and swollen. My skin is the colour of dishwater. I'm expanding and fading away at the same time.

I open a cabinet and my make-up bag spills into the bathroom sink, bronze powder exploding across the porcelain surface and onto the floor. My breathing becomes heavier and I wipe the sink clean with my hands, using my thumbnail to prise off a clump of hardened toothpaste.

I want to go back to bed and wake up somewhere else. Dip my head beneath the covers and drift into another life.

There's a gentle knock at the door. I open it and Scout is standing there.

'I need a wee-wee.'

I hoist her onto the seat and nuzzle her neck. She smells of washing powder and milk. She flinches and gently pushes me away, scanning my face, looking like she has something to say but can't form the words.

I turn away because I don't want to infect her with my sadness. I don't want this to be something she talks about in years to come in a wood-panelled office where professional empaths charge by the hour.

As she gets up and washes her hands, I close the toilet seat and sit down on the lid and the blackness falls over my vision, flashes of light dance across my eyelids. The seat is cold, Scout is there, I need to get up.

I walk her into our bedroom, where Johno is sitting in bed, scrolling the news on his phone. He looks at me and sits up straighter.

'You're up early.'

'Scout needed milk.'

My face feels still, solid, and I don't care how it looks. I'm talking to him, but I'm not there. Like there's an emptiness behind my skin and I can only see the edges of myself. Like I am two metres back, watching it all from behind.

'There's been more stuff online.'

He nods, shrugs a little, pulls Scout up onto the bed.

'I told you, you've got to ignore it. Have a day off social and they'll get bored and go away.'

I turn towards the wardrobe and move around clothes I have no intention of wearing. I can't take his fixes, I just need someone to sit in the darkness with me, instead of pointing at a ladder when I don't have limbs to climb.

I keep my voice steady, my back turned to him.

'Maybe you could take Scout today.'

'OK, sure, I can do the morning run.'

'Great.'

'But I have a meeting this afternoon.'

'Great.'

'So, I can't do pick-up.'

'No.'

I move clothes from side to side, sliding them along the rail, jumpsuits and maxi dresses and jeans and sweaters, colour everywhere, a multicoloured camouflage for all my failings.

'Are you OK, Lo?'

I keep my voice flat, and tell him, 'I'm fine.'

33

DYLAN

My phone is glowing and it's making me strong. It's like it's charging me with every tiny red heart: eighty-five comments, 3,500 new followers, dozens of private messages.

@Motherofdingbat$ 'I want you to know how brave you are.'

They know that I'm right and that I've done something good. It makes my arms feel hard and makes by belly feel tight, like there's something strong at the core of me.

I flick to Lo's feed and the picture of us is gone. Good. I breathe out, feel a little safer. Every second my face and name were there I was exposed. She showed me to 112,000 people and it felt like a 'wanted' poster. Like she was sticking me up for him to see.

@Of{Course}SheDid 'What she's done is appalling, and I hope you and your son are safe.'

Noah is dressed and his hair is brushed, so I stand by the door, ready to lead him into the world.

The paring knife is in the kitchen drawer. I put my jacket on and stop.

I feel safer now the picture is down.

I feel safer now thousands of women are with me.

There's no way he could have seen it.

But maybe, just in case, I take the knife, slip it in my jacket pocket.

We will not run away again.

I will not take Noah from the best place we have ever been.

@hopingwaiting247 *'I'm so proud of you.'*

'Right, Noh, let's go.'

I open the door to take my boy to school. We trot down the stairs and, at the bottom, I stop.

There's no way JD could have seen the post.

And even if he did see it, even if he was one of those 112,000, he might find the school, but he won't find the address.

I put my hand on the latch, but just for a second it feels like he will be there anyway, somehow smiling, waiting. Like I will open the door and he will grin.

Where you been, Dilly?

And he will want to take this boy he's never met, and he will want to own me one last time.

Except now all these women are watching.

They are watching because they care and they will protect me against men like JD and women like Lo.

And maybe he doesn't even care anymore.

Maybe I'm lucky and he really is dead.

I open the door and the day is bright. We step out and breathe

the air. I look around and the street is quiet, just us on it.

'Come on, Noah.'

I hold his hand, hold my head up. I am safe, because all these women are looking out for me and I have a little army in my phone.

As we walk, I flick to Influenza.

They are savaging Lo and there are thousands of them: she is a plagiarist and a thief, she is exploiting the vulnerable, she is aiding an abuser.

And then a new one, right on top.

CantillyAce says: Oh, hold on! I've just realised the woman she posted about is Dylan Rayne. I was at school with her. Believe me, she is NOT who she says she is.

34

LO

I kiss the top of Scout's head, kiss Johno's cheek, the front door clicks shut and I breathe in, pulling desperate air into my lungs.

Then I step back into the living room and sink into cushions moulded to the shape of my body. My phone is hot to touch. I need to know what's being said, and what to do, because I'm underwater, clasping at sand.

With each comment comes adrenaline. A little charge of, 'they might be on my side', or a little current of, 'this one is coming for me'.

There's a knock at the door and I slowly get up. The postman's face is hidden behind metallic foil packages in his arms. One is addressed to Scout and I wonder why they didn't address it to me.

'Thank you.'

I pile the packages on the floor in the hall and close the door, shivering at the chill of the air outside. I take a sip of stale squash from Scout's dinosaur cup and start writing a DM to Dyl.

'I don't know what has happened or why you felt publicly addressing me was the only way to tell me how you felt. I never intended to hurt you or harm you, I hope – and I think – you know that. I'm devastated I put you in danger. That I put Noah in danger. I never would have done that knowingly. You told me your ex was dead, Dylan. I understand if you aren't going to speak to me again, but you know I'm not what they're saying. I'm human, I'm a person, I'm here, not out there.'

I read it and delete it, fearing she might take my words out of context, post them for baying crowds, hungry for the next episode.

Jenn calls, her face cuts through my screen and I ignore it. There's another knock at the door and I ignore it. Johno's face cuts through the screen and I ignore it. I curl up, pull a cushion over my body, flick to Influenza comments.

What I hate is how she pretends to be better than everyone else.

If she really cared, she'd give everything she's earned to period poverty.

She is an abuser.

I flick to my Insta DMs.

'I'm so disappointed in you.'

'You've really let me down.'

'Do better.'

A text from Jenn.

'*Love. Been trying to call, I need to hear your voice! I'm afraid Etisk want to cancel our contract, so no need for any new content. It might just be a pause, but saves you work for now! And WeAreFemForm have pulled their whole campaign for everyone. But don't worry, I'm sure they'll be back!*'

I flick to WhatsApp and there's a list of green circles with little numbers in them, a little scoreboard of all the friendships I've ignored.

Thousands of women hate me, and it's all because of her lies.

My income is disappearing, and it's all because of her lies.

I tried to help her, to lift her up, and she has destroyed me.

And I won't let her get away with it.

So I flick back to Instagram and start writing.

This is my last post. I can't live like this, because it's not living. No one can hate me more than I hate myself right now. I know my faults, because I live with them every day. I came here to be honest about motherhood, but I've become a character in a play, a pantomime villain being screamed off stage. But I am not that. I'm human, I'm fallible, I'm flawed and I'm truly sorry for the pain I've caused. I want to apologise to every woman who saw the WeAreFemForm ads and felt traumatised by my blindness to a world I knew nothing about and shouldn't have been speaking of. I'm so truly sorry. But where is the line? I wake up every morning waiting for abuse from anonymous avatars. My relationship, my life, my daughter, are all free game because I 'put myself out there'. I did, that's my crime. I'm a blight, a bloody spot that needs to be erased. So I'll cancel myself to save anyone else having to. But there's one thing I can't stand for and that is lies. I did not intentionally steal the words of @one__day__soon, and I did not know anything about her former partner. How could I, when she told me, like she told everyone, including her son, that he was dead?

I upload the caption with a blank grey image, and my phone lights up.

35

DYLAN

Noah tugs at my hand and I ignore him.

'Mummy . . .'

> **CantillyAce says:** Dylan and I were at prep school together. Yes –
> PREP school. It cost three grand a term. Trust me, she's not the
> poor single 'mama' you have bought into. You are supporting a
> narcissistic liar on the make. Her dad was a stockbroker.

My head drifts and Noah tugs at my hand again.

'Mummy, it's time to go.'

I look down and half his class have gone in and I let his little
hand slip out of mine and watch him walk away, and then I'm
alone on the concrete with thousands of women who don't
know me and one who clearly does.

> **CantillyAce says:** The Wrythe Prep School. I saw her every day,
> right up to finishing at 13.
> **Chimichangingrooms says:** No WAY.
> **CantillyAce says:** She was a proper mean girl, too. She always
> knew how to get her way.

Filharminar says: So, it's all lies?

CantillyAce says: Wouldn't surprise me. You can't trust a word she says.

I feel light and I want to sit down.

I don't even know who this is.

I didn't know any Cantilly anything at school.

And I left at thirteen because my dad killed himself and we ran out of money, you nasty cow.

A message pings through on Instagram.

@hopingwaiting247 *'Hey Dylan. Just so you know, they're saying some weird things about you on Influenza. Sorry, I'm sure it's rubbish, I just thought you should know.'*

I go back to Influenza and the comments keep coming.

Cumbulousclouding says: I always knew she was lying.

Onatop says: It just always felt a bit too much, like she was trying to prove how poor she was.

LeilaLeila says: What a scammer! Probably keeps a crate of Verve just out of the shot whenever she takes a picture!

I look up and the caretaker is ready to close the gate. There's just me in this grey concrete space, all the kids are inside, all the parents have run away, and this little playground suddenly feels much bigger, like it's an open field and I'm miles from the edges. Like it's all boggy and my feet are stuck and no one can help me out.

The caretaker smiles and waves his keys.

'Come on,' he says. 'You're free!'

I walk towards him and get a new notification.

I've been tagged by Lo.

I walk through the gate, read the post, and it feels like someone is stirring a ladle through my belly.

Oh, Jesus, Lo.

Why are you doing this?

Why do you hate me so much?

36

LO

It is DISGUSTING that you have OUTED another woman. You are DISGUSTING.

You sold out a long time ago, Lo, so how do you expect people to buy this?

Long-term follower here. Appalled you're throwing a vulnerable woman under the bus. This is becoming the darkest version of he-says, she-says.

Did you ever stop and wonder, in your little Hague blue haven, WHY a woman might say her partner was dead?

You're playing with someone's life.

37

DYLAN

I'm standing in the street and the hate comes like waves, sucking me down, crashing on top of me.

Just one post and Lo makes the ocean surge.

I go to Instagram and they say I lied.

@Wheresmychips?

You know what happens when you make up domestic abuse? Real women who are really suffering don't get believed. You have harmed them as sure as if you hit them yourself.

@Fl!ngo76

She's basically a thief. She's stolen the focus from real victims.

@Belty[A]ishling

Private school, stockbroker dad, but that's not enough for you, is it? You've got to get more fame and attention by playing poor.

I go to Influenza and I have my own thread: 'Dylan makes it Rayne lies!'

SomeFakeUserName says: I know this is terrible, but it's a bit ironic that someone with such a hittable face would have to lie about abuse.

AllyFromTheAlley says: I just wish she'd at least have the decency to feel ashamed and go away.

DanniTheDisruptor says: What kind of sick bitch tells her boy his dad's dead? I don't care what he did, her son deserves to know his dad is alive. Filthy lying cow should have her kid taken off her.

They are talking so I can hear, but they have no faces, just a blankness where a face should be, and there are thousands of them.

I go back to Instagram and it's full of DMs and they hate me and my heart beats faster.

I tap Influenza and I slide my thumb down the screen and I am scum and my heart rattles like it might stop.

I slide my thumb again, standing in the street like a little beggar girl.

Oh, Dilly.
You're such a fuck-up.

I walk home and slide my thumb down the screen and I'm a horrible mother whose child should be taken away.

I stand in our flat and slide my thumb and I'm a fraud who is silencing real women in need.

I collect Noah from school and slide my thumb and when my son finds out I lied about his dad, he will be mentally scarred for life.

I make him a baked potato with tomato chunks on top and open the mail and Consolidated Finance Services regret to inform me that I have defaulted on my monthly plan and if payment is not made within seven days I will incur a fee of £124 and may face criminal proceedings.

I put Noah in the bath and slide my thumb and someone wonders if what I've done counts as psychological abuse and maybe they should tell the school.

And then it's 2.00 a.m. and Noah is asleep and I'm in bed, but even when I close my eyes, the messages are still there.

It's like there's a blue-white glow fixed behind my eyelids and when I try to shut my eyes, it fills with their words and their tags. So I reach for my phone and Instagram. I swipe down my thumb.

> **@trainwreck\in\motion**
> *You have done harm to every woman who really suffers because now they will never be believed.*
> **@hopingwaiting247**
> *She doesn't care. She is a cancer.*

I block them all, make my account private, but by daybreak there are more on Influenza, thousands more, enraged because I'm running away.

> **Kalabash says:** Have you seen that Dylan Rayne has gone? Blocked everyone? Just proves it was all lies. She's probably at her country retreat!

And then it's 8.00 a.m. and Noah is eating porridge and I am ignoring him and my heart feels tired, like it has been sprinting all night and might soon need to stop.

The flat feels smaller and dirtier. This is the best place I've ever had and it's a shithole and I'm not fit to care for my boy.

I have lied to him in the most terrible way, and one day he will find out and hate me forever.

Like thousands of women hate me now, because they think I lied about being poor.

And it doesn't matter what's true.

The world thinks I'm foul and should lose my son.

And it's all because of her.

38
LO

It's 8.30 a.m. and Johno leans over the bed to peck my cheek before taking Scout to school.

'Did you sleep?'

'A bit.'

'Good. You OK for pick-up today?'

'Yes.'

He leaves with Scout, and as the door closes, I sob.

They came all night and all morning, too. And when I close my eyes, there is a weight across my lungs like I have to inhale hard to get the air in, and even when I turn off my phone, I can still hear their voices.

I shut it down and put it in a drawer, but I can still hear their whispering. So I go back and turn it on, so I can know exactly what they're saying.

The moment anyone challenges you, you find a vulnerable woman to shit on. It is sick. You are sick.

And it is. It is so sick and so am I.

I made a mistake, did a terrible ad and I just needed her help.

But she turned them on me when I needed her most.

After all I've done for her, after I got her started and gave her a voice, she stirred them up and sent them my way.

So I had to defend myself.

Because this is all her fault.

39

DYLAN

I've got 1,412 new follower requests on Instagram. More women wanting to watch the circus. I flick to Influenza to see the ways in which women hate me, and they hate me because I had a life that's different to what they expected.

I look at my laptop, ChatTeam open but ignored, and flick to my emails and there's one from H2-Oh. They are concerned about my 'decreased call volume', and 'commitment to my sales affiliate status'.

And then a call.

A landline I don't recognise and an urgent pulsing green symbol on my phone. I tap, and there's a familiar voice.

'DYLAN?'

'Yes, is that Callum?'

'It IS!'

'Are you OK?'

'Yes, but more importantly, how are you?'

'I'm OK.'

His voice is less sure now than the other day, a little quieter.

'I just wanted to check in, off the back of some of the online stuff.'

'Oh.'

'Looks a little extreme, some of it.'

'Yes, it's been a bit . . .'

And I don't know what to say, because it's been a bit like nothing I've felt before.

'But you're keeping well?'

Debt collectors are coming for me, thousands of women hate me, I have told a heinous lie to the boy I love more than anything on Earth.

'I'm fine.'

'Good, because I've been wanting to catch up.'

'Yes . . .'

'We've been having a little think here.'

'Yes.'

'And there are some concerns about what's being said.'

'What do you mean?'

'Well, there's quite a lot online and . . . have you seen the *Mail* this morning?'

'No, what's happened?'

The prickles rush up me, little stabs across the skin of my neck.

'It's small. Just the website, and I'm sure it won't grow. It's just that . . .'

I open the *Mail*'s website on my laptop, scroll past dozens of stories, and there it sits, halfway down, a tiny little square with my face and Lo's side by side.

'Influencer Dylan Rayne Accused of "Faking Poverty" and "Lying to Her Son" That His Dad was DEAD'.

I feel my knees go empty, like someone has scooped out the bones and the flesh of me, and I sit on the kitchen floor and feel the prickles on my chest and the itching on the ridges on my arms.

'. . . Thing is, Dylan, it's just that we do now face a slight credibility issue and some negative associations. Of course, your book is fiction – and I still love it, don't get me wrong, that murder at the end is so wonderfully detailed – it's just that—'

'What, Callum, please tell me what . . .'

'We'd like to take a little pause before getting the contracts over, just to let all of this unpleasantness pass.'

His words hang, my phone is limp in my hand, and I hold my mouth open, searching for words that don't come.

'But . . .'

'BECAUSE, though they say there is no such thing as bad publicity, some publicity really can do harm.'

'It's not true.'

'No, of course, and horrible to be caught up in.'

Except it is true. I went to a posh school until my dad ran out of money and threw himself in front of a train. I lied to my boy, told him his dad was dead, because I never want JD to find us and if he does, I might have to stab him in the heart.

'So, Dylan, what we're thinking here is that maybe we can come back next year. Maybe springtime, or summer, or so. Have a little think then. I do hope you understand.'

And I've got nothing to say, except, 'OK.'

'Great, well, all the best.'

And then he's gone, and I feel the room get smaller. Like a cloud shifts over the winter sun and the air gets greyer.

He's gone because he doesn't want me anymore.

Just like Dad didn't want me.

Even JD doesn't want me.

Because no one wants me, except an army of women staring in, ready to burn the witch.

And I want to know why Lo gets to keep her nice life and mine gets taken away.

I want to know why she gets to win.

Why she has so much more than me.

She has so much more than me, and still she wants to take all I have.

But I will not allow it, because this is the best life we've ever had.

I go to the counter and get the paring knife.

I crouch on my knees and prepare myself.

Because it'll be important to move quickly.

40
LO

I put my long puffa coat over my pyjamas and tuck them into my wellies and step into the rain. Only a slither of striped fabric at the shin gives it away.

As I walk, I clutch my phone with one hand and the other finds an old ibuprofen packet in a pocket corner and I rub my finger over the empty pill sockets. My hood is up and I shrink into the warmth, realising I've forgotten Scout's snack. It's too late to turn back; I'm already late. I imagine her standing alone in the school line and my heart aches: a girl looking out for her mum and wondering why she isn't there again. Nausea creeps in and I realise I haven't eaten breakfast or lunch, haven't tasted water. I need food and the baby needs to eat. I find myself holding my stomach like it's a soother. Like the purity of a foetus inside can somehow erase the world outside. I pull out my phone and notifications flood the screen, droplets of rain pooling on the cracked and splintered surface. A notification from Babycentre.com tells me my baby is the size of a peppercorn and has begun to develop its brain, spinal cord and heart.

There's a missed call from school and I put the phone in my

pocket, block the noise for a moment. I'll be there soon, they can tell me anything then.

I keep my head down against the drizzle and walk faster. My body carries me but someone else is driving. My eyes hurt and my stomach feels tangled. It's bad for the baby, but the baby won't live anyway. Babies won't live in me because my uterus doesn't work and Scout was a one-time miracle.

I reach the playground and it's almost empty – all the other parents have been and gone – and I see two small figures standing side by side in the greyness under a rainbow umbrella held by Ms Carole. As I get closer, I can see it's Scout and Noah and a shiver rises up me, freezing my feet for half a pace. I look around, dreading the sight of Dyl, but she's not there, so I turn back to the teacher to get this done as quickly as possible.

'Sorry I'm late.'

My voice is muffled from within my coat. I grab Scout's hand and turn to leave.

'Sorry, one thing.'

Ms Carole sounds urgent. I wonder if this moment will give Dyl time to arrive. I feel sick and want to keep walking.

'Yes?'

'Have you had contact with Noah's mum today?'

She scans my face. Does she know? Does she know what they're saying about me?

'Um . . .'

'We've tried contacting her and she hasn't responded. She has you on the list as the next person to call.'

I'm still clasping Scout's hand.

'What do you mean?'

'If a child hasn't been collected after twenty minutes, our protocol is to call a parent or guardian. The office called you and your husband about Scout, but Noah's mother hasn't replied.'

'She's probably coming.'

'And you're the only other person on her list.'

'But I'm not next of kin.'

'It isn't always. If there's no family. And I believe you'd both agreed?'

And we had, but that was before.

The rain starts to spit a little harder and she looks at me as I look at Noah, huddled next to her leg to take shelter under her umbrella.

'So what does this mean?'

Ms Carole lowers her voice. 'After an hour, if there has been no contact, then the protocol is that we contact social services and, eventually, the police.'

Then maybe that's OK. Maybe they can take him.

'I'm sure she's coming.'

But as I say it, I wonder if maybe she isn't.

'But what do social services do?'

'Well, ultimately, and this never really happens, they might have to find emergency accommodation. But that's very rare. Usually if there's a problem, friends or family step in.'

Noah looks up at us and his face, like Ms Carole's, is frowning. Scout looks up at me, rain splattering her hood, and Ms Carole looks at me hopefully.

I am the name on Dyl's list.

I am her person for emergencies, because she has no one else. She is alone and has no one to trust with her child, except a school mum she hates.

I can't leave him here.

'OK, well, yes, I can take him. Come on, Noah, I'm going to take you to your house.'

I say this as though it's exciting, even though I feel chilled that I am with her son.

Scout chimes in. 'Like a playdate?'

'Sort of.'

I hold both their hands tightly and we walk out of the red gates as the caretaker closes them behind us. I have no more fight left.

I'll take what she throws at me for turning up with her son.

41
LO

Noah walks a little in front of me, confidently striding home. He's four, but he looks like a little man, just missing a trench coat and briefcase.

'I'm so impressed you know the way home, Noah,' I say, trying to break the nervous silence.

He shrugs. 'It's a straight line.'

And he is right. Maybe we underestimate them at every turn? They're just adults trapped in small bodies.

I call Dyl again, but she ignores me, so when we get to her door, I ring her bell, but it's silent.

'You have to knock,' says Noah.

So I knock, but nothing.

I stand back and feel sick as I wait for a rumble of feet down the stairs, or her face at the window, and know that I will soon have to look at the woman who has done this to me.

But she doesn't come and I knock again.

I knock a third time and then a fourth, each one more urgent, but nothing.

Where are you, Dylan, and what game are you playing?

I look down at her son and see worry creeping across his face and Scout's.

'Well, then, maybe we'll have tea at our place? I'm sure she'll be back soon, Noah. She probably had a meeting and got stuck on the Tube. How about sausages?'

'OK.'

He smiles, but it is a smile for me, not for him.

42
LO

The key turns and Johno walks in, and I look up from my phone. It feels hot in my hand, overworked from telling me the worst things I already know about myself.

'It's eight o'clock,' I tell him.

His face drops. It sinks because I weary him.

'I know. I told you I had a meeting.'

He smells of beer.

'In a pub?'

'No, I went to the pub afterwards and I sat on my own and had one pint and read the paper like an old man.'

'Sorry.'

I say it tightly and he sighs.

'It's fine. Hi, Noah.'

The kids are silent, bathed in the blue glow from the TV. Noah says hello and Scout looks up, then turns back to *The Secret Life of Pets*.

'Is Dyl here?'

'No.'

He frowns.

'Where is she?'

I get up and whisper, 'We don't know. She didn't pick him up. She's not answering my calls. She didn't answer the door. That's why I wanted you home.'

I didn't need the last part. He didn't know. It feels like there's so much he doesn't know.

'Well, I'm here now.' He's sullen, but then he tries to make a joke. 'Although this really isn't what I meant when I said we should have another kid.'

I don't reply. I go upstairs, pull on warmer clothes and leave.

The rain has eased when I return to Dyl's. There's a steady sheen now. More than spitting, less than a downpour, just a chilled dampness all over me. I bang the door again, but nothing. I turn to my phone, the battery is low, but I get a flurry of notifications – little taps on the shoulder from a mob that wants me gone.

I call Dylan again, but she doesn't reply.

Maybe she's drunk. Maybe she's been in a car crash. Maybe she's run away.

I bang louder and call up to her front window.

'Dyl!'

It feels wrong even saying her name, like it's something else that's not mine to use, and I bang loudly again. Nothing. And then a rattle of a chain and the click of a lock.

'Hello?'

It's a little old woman I've not seen before, and she's not sure about me.

'Hi. Does Dyl live here?'

'Yes. Upstairs.'

'Can I go up?'

She hesitates. I take down my hood so she can see me better.

'I'm Lo. My daughter is at school with Dyl's son and she didn't collect him today.'

She looks worried now.

'Where is Noah?'

'At our house. Maybe I can try her door?'

She nods and pushes the door aside and there's a dark staircase with a worn black carpet.

'Is there a light?'

She shakes her head. 'Not working.'

I go up the stairs and she waits at the bottom, wedging open the front door to give some light, but it's still too dark to see.

'Does she have a bell?'

I look downstairs at the old lady and she shrugs, so I knock on the door. I bang five times with my knuckles, a friendly little rhythm. There's no reply and no movement.

I knock again, three times now in loud, plain beats.

Nothing again.

I look down at the old woman.

'Have you seen her today?'

She shakes her head.

'Wait. I have key.'

She goes back into her flat and I knock again.

The old lady climbs the stairs slowly, hand on the rail, and passes the key to me three steps from the top, stiff as she moves.

I can't see the lock, so I pull out my phone. Small shards of glass catch in my thumb as I turn on the torch. I find the lock, the paint around it chipped and flaked by hundreds of stabbed efforts to get in.

The lock turns and it's dark inside.

I take a step through, feel around for a light switch.

And then I fall to the floor.

43

LO

The blood is in a pool and the old lady is crying her name.

'Dyl-AN! Dyl-AN!'

She says it in a strange way, with the emphasis on the end, and it's all I can hear and my knees are damp. The blood is coming through my leggings and I'm holding up her left wrist, folding down her hand against her forearm and the dark, wet line.

I am holding it and pressing it, but her face is a strange colour. Her skin is grey and I have her arm up, but now blood is running down her skin in little rivers. Little lines crawling down and curving and turning over old ridges I'd never seen before, horizontal scars crossing over all the way from wrist to elbow, and I don't know what to do.

I pull down a tea towel and tie it around her wrist, but it soaks so quickly. I take off my coat and wrap it around her body, trying to work with one hand while holding up her arm. I lay the coat across her and try to wrap it underneath. Try to swaddle this thin body to keep it warm and the old lady says:

'Ambulance!'

And I say, 'Yes, now.'

But then she's giving the address and I see she is not talking to me but talking on my phone to a 999 operator.

She is saying, 'Stem bleeding. Apply pressure. Pressing! Pressing!'

And I say, 'Yes, I am.' But I don't think it's enough. I don't think it's enough and I don't think I can do this and I'm letting her die.

She is dying now because of me and because I am not doing enough to help her because I don't know what to do.

And then the old lady has towels and one of them is Noah's because it is red and yellow and has Superman on it and maybe he wears it like a cape when he's had a bath. Wears it like a cape and runs around and won't put on his pyjamas and now it's tied tight around her wrist and how the fuck could you do this, Dylan? How the fuck could you do this to him?

The old lady is saying her name again but softer this time. She's stroking her head and saying her name like she's trying to wake up a little girl.

'Dylan? Can you hear me, Dylan?'

But there's no response.

And we stay like that for a while.

I press the towel tight and hold up her arm and the old lady strokes her head and says her name again and again, but Dylan doesn't move because she's dying.

And the old lady looks at me and we're both scared because we know that this is it.

She will die in our arms and go cold while we hold her.

'Hello? Ambulance service.'

'Yes, here!'

They come in and fill the room. They both look large and strong, this man and woman. Their clothes are big and green and yellow and they have pockets and belts full of equipment and a case like a toolkit for broken people.

'OK, just step aside please.'

They are calm and quick and I sit back in the corner and the old woman moves away and begins to cry. She weeps in the corner and I realise that I've been crying, too. My eyes feel empty and salt crusts my lashes and my voice hurts, so maybe I shouted, too. I sit there and watch and beside Dylan is a phone with blood-red fingerprints on the screen.

The paramedics attach proper bandages to her wrist and wrap these tight and ask us her name, then they say it firmly.

'Dylan? Can you hear me? We're paramedics, Dylan, and we're going to take you to hospital.'

Then the woman paramedic turns to me.

'Do you know if she's taken anything? Any tablets, drugs, alcohol?'

I shake my head and shrug because I don't know.

Then they have blankets around her and she is tied to a stretcher and my coat is on the floor.

And as they lift her, the woman says, 'Right. Would anyone like to come with us?'

44
LO

I am strapped to a green chair and the sirens are wailing like they're in pain. The woman is talking to Dyl and shouting information at the man as he drives and talks into his radio. We lurch and move too fast and it feels like we might crash, and I can see Dyl's fragile body bounce a little as we hit a pothole.

My face crumples as the woman frowns and goes back to her work, talking to the man behind the wheel and then talking to Dyl.

'Dylan, can you tell me if you can hear anything at all?'

But Dylan doesn't speak.

'Will she be OK?' I ask, my voice cracking.

I ask because I want her to lie to me and say that she will be fine.

'We'll do everything we can.'

45

DYLAN

DanniTheDisruptor says: She should have her kid taken off her, filthy lying cow.

46

LO

It's been four hours. This is where they bring the ones who didn't make it and the ones who still might not, and I can feel my heart shudder.

A man in overalls is leaving with his wife and a freshly bandaged arm, and the plastic floor is flecked with rubber marks from wheels and trainers and rushing bodies.

The fluorescent lights bleach my skin, like I'm a lab rat in a test. Jets of air pour out of a vent above me and the heat is breeding germs and my heart thumps and I think I might be sick. I tap my phone, but my phone is useless, the battery dead, the screen smashed.

I twist my hair with my thumb and index finger and strands slide away into my palm. I pull gently again and another strand comes and somehow it's soothing me away from Dyl's wrists and the blood pooling on the floor, the blood on my clothes.

She's somewhere in this building, this place where our kids were both born, and either she's dead already or they're pouring blood into her, filling up the cracks. I wonder whose blood it is. If it was an old man who died in his sleep, or a donor trying to do the right thing.

There was so much blood on that floor and I wonder what the police will ask.

There's blood on the knees of my leggings and my coat, blood on my hoodie, and my hands are raw from scrubbing them in the toilet.

The police haven't come yet, but the mob soon will.

When they learn she has died, they will say I made her do it, and I should die, too. And they are right.

Maybe I should give them what they want, because at least then I wouldn't have to hear them.

My heart is so empty it feels like it might have stopped. Like I've been emptied. Like someone has scraped out my muscles and marrow, and I so badly want to sleep.

'Hello, are you with Ms Rayne?'

The nurse is Scottish and her voice is soft. She has cropped, brown hair and sounds like she cares about everything. I nod at her.

'Sorry you've had such a long wait, would you like to come through?'

'Is she OK?'

'I don't know. The doctor will come in a while.'

'But is she alive?'

She stops and turns around.

'Oh, yes. But she's very poorly.'

'But she will live?'

'The doctor will come in a while.'

We turn through corridors where the lights get brighter, a dirty yellow washing all over us. But this nurse walks quickly and the movement shifts my heart.

Because if Dyl's alive, she can blame me.

She can tell them all that I made her do it.

My knees buckle.

My hands touch the floor.

'Oh, dear.'

The nurse puts her hands on me and I want to cry. I want to be cared for. Noises come out of me and tears fall from my face.

'All right, let's get you sitting down.'

She lifts me onto a chair.

'Now, did you twist anything?'

I shake my head and my shoulders heave.

'It's OK,' she says. 'She's getting the best care.'

She holds my hands and I want to feel some warmth around me and from nowhere I lean forward and I hug her. I wrap my arms around her and she holds me like I'm a giant toddler with a scraped knee.

'There, there, it's all right.'

She is warm and she is soft and it feels in this moment like she is the only person on earth who cares for me. So I don't let her go until she pulls back to look at me.

'Let me get you some water and some tea and a comfy seat outside the ICU. They've got the good biscuits, too.'

I wake up on a beige-pink plastic chair in the corridor outside the ICU.

The Scottish nurse convinced them to let me use the desk phone to call Johno, and they watched me cry as I told him. The kids were long asleep by then, but I don't think I've slept for long.

The tall Victorian windows here have no blinds, and a grey-white light fills every space. It sits in the room, like a pale cloud has entered the building. My neck aches and my spine is stiff, but it's still more sleep than I've had in days.

'Would you like a cup of tea?'

A new nurse has appeared and is holding a steaming mug that I take without speaking.

'The consultant will be along later to speak to you.'

She turns to go and I call out, 'Wait!'

It comes out too loud and she looks shocked, like I'm calling for service, and a frown comes over her as she turns back to face me.

'Sorry, I just . . . I wonder if you might have a phone charger?'

'I do, actually.'

She states this calmly; looks at me like I'm a petulant teen who has forgotten how to say please and thank you.

'Could I borrow it, just for a minute, please? There are people I need to talk to.'

She looks at me, sees something pathetic, pleading; the woman with someone else's blood on her clothes.

'Of course, I was just using it myself.'

She reaches into her pocket and pulls one out, hands it to me.

'Bring it back when you're done. There's a socket just there.'

She points to the wall, just above the floor, and I go to my knees and stab in the three pins, push the other end of the wire into my phone, turn it on, hold it and hope as the nurse walks silently away. Very slowly, there is a flicker of life, my apps beneath a web of shattered plastic, distorted, and all I want to know is what they're saying.

On Influenza they're saying I am disgusting. They're saying I harm women and I lie and cheat and exploit.

On Instagram they're saying I am an abuser. They're saying I gaslight.

And then in my direct messages one says: '*I can help you.*'

My thumb stops, I peer closer, edge the message up and down, make the words move around my damaged screen as

I read through the splinters and cracks. Another anonymous woman.

> 'I can help you. I can see what's happening, and I've followed you for some time, and I can help you.'

I read the words and I desperately need them to be true but don't know how they can be.

> 'I can help you to understand what you have done to your "friend". Because when I saw her face on your feed, I recognised her straight away. I recognised it because it was shown to me many times, by a man named James Dempsey. When he wanted to tell me I was fat, he would show me her picture. When he wanted to tell me I was old, he would show it to me again. When he wanted to tell me I wasn't good enough, he would show me what he once had. And I was with him for two years, because just for a little while, every now and then, he made me feel wanted and loved. And I want to help you understand that, how a woman can be so lost, because I don't think you do. I used to love what you did, because it made me laugh when not much does, but I don't love it anymore. I want you to understand that whatever she has done, you have made your friend very afraid. You will have made her very afraid that he will come back and do whatever he did before all over again. Because when I wouldn't do what he told me, he would lock me in my own flat. He would steal my money and slap my head. He would lie to my friends and tell me I was stupid and I guess he did all those things to her, too. But I want you to tell her that she doesn't need to be scared anymore. Because when he punctured my lung and broke my jaw, I wasn't scared anymore, either, I was angry. I was angry with him, and with me, for letting him do it and that day I said that he wouldn't be allowed to do it ever again, to me or to anyone else. So I told the police, and I stood in a

dock, and I let him see me as I told them everything and now he's in prison for a very long time. So I want you to tell her that. And I want you to know the fear you have made her feel. Because even though he is bricked up and behind bars, I still see him everywhere I go. I see him in every shop, round every corner, because a man like that will never be gone. I wanted to help you understand that, because I don't think you do.'

I hold my phone down, feel my eyes redden at the edges, sit on the floor to try to understand what I've just read. What I've done to Dyl.

There's a voice over my shoulder.

'This is Mr Khan, the consultant dealing with your friend.'

Beside the nurse is a tall man, maybe my age, and I stand to look at him. He has on dark blue chinos and a pale blue Oxford shirt, and without a stethoscope he could be one of the accountants that works with Johno.

He speaks very softly, like I might be about to become a patient too.

'Dylan is awake and she is calm and we've just finished our morning checks.'

He stops to let the information settle, but he does it in a way that doesn't invite me to interrupt.

'She cut her radial artery, causing severe haemorrhage, and by the time you found her, she was in hypovolemic shock from the loss of blood. This is what caused her to lose consciousness and probably meant she felt quite cold when you found her.'

'Yes.'

He gives me a kind smile.

'That can be very worrying.'

I just nod and stare down at the floor and see he has bright white trainers and red socks.

'We gave her a lot of blood over the first few hours and sutured the laceration. Her toxicology report was clean. She may have some impaired movement for a while, but we don't believe there is nerve damage, so we don't expect that to be permanent.'

'She won't die?'

He smiles.

'Not today. She's in good hands. And, I should say as well, with this kind of laceration, there isn't much time to act. A few hours at most before the blood loss becomes too significant and organs fail. Your intervention was key.'

Yes, my intervention was key. You have no idea how key it was.

'So when can she go home?'

The smile goes now, and the soft voice returns.

'In treatments of this nature, it is not just a case of returning home, I'm afraid. Physically, the main job has been done and she'll be able to leave ICU tomorrow, I expect. But not to go home. She will go to a psychiatric ward for evaluation.'

'For how long?'

'It's hard to say. She's calm now, but we will need to monitor that. At least a week, usually two, sometimes longer. She has been asking about her son. Provisions will need to be made for his care.'

He looks at me and waits.

'What provisions?'

'Usually family, a guardian. If not family, then trusted friends. Otherwise, social services.'

And I wonder what that means: emergency fostering with strangers? Noah in an institution? A kids' home with passcodes for the doors and fire extinguishers on the walls and everything made wipe-clean? And what kids will be there with him, and what he will think every night as he falls asleep.

'She has asked to see you.'

*

The nurse ushers me to her room, tucking her charger in her pocket and talking over her shoulder as we walk.

'I'll have to ask you not to leave anything with her. No hair clips, belts.'

She opens the door like a compère unveiling a new show. The bed sheets are starched and brilliant white, a heart monitor bleeps and Dyl has a thick bandage around her wrist.

She looks even smaller now, like a newborn sparrow in a pristine white nest. Her skin is as pale as her sheets, her eyes yellow at the edges. Her black roots and bleached hair tangled across the pillow and her lips look cracked.

She's alive.

Her heart is drawing green lines on a screen.

The nurse steps out and closes the door, leaving us alone.

Dyl looks at me and I'm rooted to the spot. My chest starts to heave and my face clenches, eyes shut, hot tears waiting behind the lids. I can't move, I can't help. I can only stand here, like a child that knows it's done something terrible.

She's blank and still and looks at me.

I breathe back hard, suck everything in, exhale and wipe my eyes.

'Where's Noah?'

Her voice is soft and crackles.

'He's safe. He's with us.'

A gasp overcomes her, but no words form and she turns her face away.

I slowly move closer and sit in the chair by her bed.

And I can see for the first time, in her short-sleeved hospital gown, all the little ridges up her arm. Little lines from a life I've misunderstood.

Her forehead crinkles, she sucks in air and fixes her face.

329

Her lips are open wide, pursed, and she cries. Her body shakes, rapid jiggles of her shoulders, and she puts her unbandaged hand over her face.

'He's OK, Dyl.'

I reach for the other hand, with its thick bandage around her wrist and palm, just her fingers free, and I stroke them.

'He was all I could think about,' she says. 'When it was getting cold, he was all I could think about.'

The sounds stab out of her. Like the air and the tears are charging forward and she can't stop them, and all I can think of is how peaceful the kids looked when I left. How warm and untroubled against the TV glare. The whorl of Noah's crown spiralling in all directions, and how he looks like Dyl, but softer, his nose rounder, his cheeks chubbier.

'He's OK, Dyl, I promise.'

I rub my thumb over her fingertips, feel the tiny furrows of our fingerprints together.

'Did he see me?'

She turns to one side to hide her face from me.

'No. It was me and your neighbour.'

There is much Noah will remember from these days, but he won't be scarred with that picture.

She blows out hard, steadies her breathing.

'I didn't mean to,' she says.

I nod, don't know what to say. She thinks I don't believe her.

'It's something I used to do,' she says, 'a long time ago, when I needed to feel something different, but I never meant to . . .'

I nod.

'I just used to do it for a little release, just a little cut. Something else to focus on. I couldn't do that to Noah. I would never leave him.'

And she heaves again, a sob forcing its way out in a gust.

'I know, Dyl. It's OK.'

'It just went too deep.'

'Yes.'

Her words come in tumbles, air gasping, tears running, like there's not enough oxygen in her to speak and let the pain out at the same time. She blows out a breath like she's being hit with a contraction, clears her throat, steadies herself, finds the hard face she had on the day we first met.

'I was drifting, and he was all I could think of, and I saw my phone there, but it was like my arms were soft and I couldn't dial.'

I stroke her hand and nod and we sit in silence, the rhythmic beep of the heart monitor punctuating the stagnant air. She turns back towards me and we look at each other properly for the first time.

'I'm so sorry,' I say, softly.

She gazes out of the window.

'I am sorry about all of it,' I say again. 'I thought it was your fault they were coming after me, but I'd already done the damage to myself.'

She nods, sighs. 'I was scared is all. About my ex. Angry about you using something I'd said.'

'I didn't even realise . . .'

She shakes her head like it's an irrelevance. Turns her face back to look at me, but she can't say anything, so I do.

'You didn't tell me about your ex.'

'No.'

'Was it bad with him?'

She sighs again, all the air flowing out like she's deflating.

'Nothing you could prove.'

'I'm so sorry, Dyl.'

She shrugs, licks her dry lips, and I pour her some water

from the plastic jug by her bed. I fill her cup and she takes it with her good hand, then I fill one for me. I want to drink it all, to fill every dried cell of my body. She looks at me.

'I've had a message,' I say.

Her eyes stay hard, like she's not listening.

'From a woman who knew him, too.'

She tenses, looks sharply at me, tries to sit up.

'What? What woman?'

'She says she went out with him, but now he's in prison. James Dempsey.'

Her eyes narrow, pupils shrink, like it's suddenly got very bright; and she looks for a second like she might fall, but she has nowhere to go. Her mouth opens, but there are no sounds.

'You can read it,' I say and hand her my phone.

She takes it, pinches at the screen with her good hand, stabs her fingers over the cracks, can't hold it with her injured hand and so sits up to rest it on her lap. She peers in and reads and very slowly the tears return and silently fall on her white bed sheet, leaving little dots of damp grey.

'Is that his name?'

She nods, closes her eyes, and a little gasp falls out of her.

'He's just been there so long,' she says. 'Been in my head for so long, and I could've stopped him, but I just ran away. Just left him out there to do it again.'

She leans back, stares up. Silent howls shudder her shoulders and they bounce up and down as her face crumples, screws her hand over her eyes, and I instinctively need to touch her, rub my palm over her shin like she's Scout after a fall, and we sit like that for a while.

'I'm sorry, Dyl, I never knew. If I'd known about him . . .'

She shakes her head, eyes wide open now, unsure what to say or do, and gives a little laugh, then a sigh.

'All this time, I didn't need to be scared.'

She's talking to the air now, looking up, and then she looks at me, relief washing over her.

'I never meant to put you in danger,' I say. 'To scare you . . .'

She shakes her head again.

'Can you send me her name?'

'She's anonymous.'

Dyl shrugs. I screen-grab as best I can, tap about my smashed screen and forward on the image of the woman's message and handle.

'It's with you.'

She nods her thanks.

'Hard to believe we were flashing our bits at each other a few weeks ago.'

And the crassness of it makes me smile.

She sighs again, exhales loudly. She is matter-of-fact once more, the top layer of tears expelled.

'We didn't have to do it,' she says.

'No.'

We didn't have to do it.

We didn't have to do any of it.

We don't have to like each other and we don't have to agree, but we don't have to destroy each other, either.

We could collect our kids and let them play and leave each other alone.

We don't need to serve each other up to faceless judgement. We don't need to join the mob or stir it up.

'The doctor says I might have to stay here.'

She says it plainly, like she's discussing train times.

'Yes. What about Noah? What should we tell him? Should he stay with us or is there someone else?'

She teases the hem of the sheet with her finger and thumb, drops her eyes, continues her monotone.

'I might speak to my mum.'

'Where is she?'

'Still down in Sutton.'

'Oh.'

'We haven't spoken in a long while, but this might be the time. She hasn't seen him for a couple of years.'

I nod, and with her lying there, her voice still and her body cloistered in white, it's like some strange confessional.

'After Dad died, it was bad between us,' she says. 'She moved on quite fast and I sort of blamed her for not seeing how sad he was.'

I nod again, let her speak.

'But you can't ever really know that,' she says, 'if someone doesn't tell you themselves.'

And it sinks into the room that she has had no one for a very long time.

'He can stay with us.'

She nods, thinks.

'Maybe a couple of nights.'

'We'll tell him it's a mega sleepover.'

'Yes.'

The air goes silent.

'Did you bring my phone?'

'No, sorry.'

'Probably best.'

A nurse pokes her head around the door.

'That's probably enough for today,' she says, with a gentle smile.

We both nod and she moves on.

I stroke Dylan's good hand.

'Can you bring Noah in?'

'Yes, of course. What should we say about what happened?'

'Maybe . . . tell him I had a fall.'

The words cling in her mouth and we stare for a moment in stillness. She looks up at me as I stand.

'Yes.'

I nod. I'll keep it vague for him. Maybe he's young enough to accept that.

Dyl raises her head.

'I wonder,' she says, 'who they all are.'

I shrug.

'Just strangers, mostly. I don't really know.'

But I know something must change. I pull my phone from my pocket, the cracked screen reflecting my face, distorting my shape, making me look alien.

'Do you think they'll keep coming for us?'

'Maybe, for a while,' I say.

She nods.

'I'm sorry, Lo.'

'I'm sorry, Dyl.'

We both smile weakly, say goodbye, and as I walk towards the door, I drop my phone in a small, locked yellow bin marked 'Sharps'.

47

JULY

DYLAN

The playground is done up like a carnival and I'm one of the first parents there.

I've got our big holdall at my feet and stand with one leg either side so no one steps on it.

There's a red-and-black bouncy castle over next to the bike shed, with big inflatable ladybird antennae flapping in the wind. A few mums have tables of food lined up against the fences and are unwrapping Cellophane and piling up paper plates or putting out little handwritten notes saying, 'Samosas 50p', or 'Fairy Cakes – Two for £1'.

Gav, the caretaker, is using a hose to fill a massive blue bucket with water next to some stocks made from old pallets. On the stocks, there's a big hole for a head and two smaller holes for arms and each plank of wood is painted a different colour of the rainbow. Next to it is a wooden A-frame board that must be older than most of the teachers here, with a hand-painted sign in a thick gloss on a flaking yellow background, done in that neat, round writing teachers do when they're trying to show kids how letters work: 'Sponge a Teacher! Three goes for £1'.

Very faintly, you can still see where old numbers were painted underneath and it looks like the price used to be 10p.

Gav swishes the hose back and forth like it will make the bucket fill faster and stares down as the sponges bob about.

I call him Gav if we speak, sometimes say hello, but we don't speak much. He introduced himself when I first came back, said he'd heard and hoped I was OK, but he doesn't smile at me anymore, just gives me this soft look, like he's trying to make his eyes all caring.

A few people said hello in those early days back.

There's a girl in Noah's class called Letitia, whose mum I kind of recognised, and on that first pick-up after my accident, with Mum there next to me holding my hand like I was a little toddler, she came up and rubbed my arm.

Just walked up and sort of leaned forward, like she didn't want to stand too close in case it scared me, and then she put her palm flat on my upper arm and said, 'It's really good to see you back.'

A couple of weeks on a psych ward and suddenly everyone wants to be mates.

I feel like they're still looking, some of them, because word gets around. Little glances in the playground, like I might suddenly top myself by the hopscotch.

But I won't.

And I wasn't trying to.

And most people have been nice.

Mum, too.

Maybe they were always there, these women, and I just needed to look for them.

The playground is filling up as the volunteer parents make the place ready. There's a jumble sale in one corner, a barbecue

337

drum smoking in another. And out of the way to one side is a big black plastic box full of old uniform bits. Frayed jumpers and trousers and skirts, donated for parents who can't afford their own. I could look for something for Noah, but our bag is already full with holiday clothes.

The chatter builds as more mums and dads fill the concrete space. There are too many of us already, with all these stalls, and they haven't even released the kids yet.

I look about and check the sky. It's nearly sunny and nearly raining, blue bits of sky and pale grey clouds being pushed along by the wind, and when the sun is set free, it feels too hot, but then things go colder, greyer, like someone is fiddling the brightness dial.

A dad stands next to me, nods. The crowd builds steadily. All these bodies huddled together, even less space because of all the clutter of a school fete.

We're being forced together, standing so close, people have to acknowledge each other. Another mum smiles, raises her eyebrows as if to say, 'here we go again,' and I smile back and pull my cardigan sleeves down over my hands.

I wouldn't have liked this crowd before, but they taught me some exercises in hospital. Ways of breathing. Ways of calming myself that don't involve a blade. I still feel the prickles, still wonder if JD might be there, but not as much.

He's in a cell, locked up, given food and a bit of exercise and a long way from me. But even if he was dead, I think he'd still be with me, just a little; a whisper in the back of my skull. Men like that stay with you long after they're gone.

But the whisper will get quieter, and most days I can breathe.

Most days I take big gulps of beautiful, grubby London air and think of my wonderful boy and the life we might still lead, and that air reaches my toes and fingertips and calms my belly and makes me glad to be here. Lucky and proud and glad.

I jolt as my leg buzzes, and reach in and pull out my phone. A crappy little Nokia with Snake and calls and not much else, where it takes five minutes to write a text.

It's Mum, sending me the address of the cottage in Whitstable again. She's on the train and will have dinner ready when we arrive, so long as we get the 4.40. I text her, '*OK*' and then add a little kiss.

We'll be there for a week, the first time we've slept under the same roof in about ten years, and she's promised to take Noah crabbing while I work.

Me nearly dying has done wonders for our relationship.

But it is strange having a mother again. Like we have to re-learn how it works and who can make what decisions. She came to the hospital on the third day and cried more than me and insisted on taking Noah, but I told her, no, Noah doesn't know you.

This week will change that.

The school bell rings and makes the parents more alert, eyes forward, waiting for their kid. Soon my boy will be in my arms, and tonight he will smell sea air for the first time and maybe his nana will read him a bedtime story.

To my left, I see Lo, making slow progress to the edge of the crowd and waiting there.

She looks good pregnant. She looks full: round but firm, every curve completely filled and she sort of glows. There's life in her skin, in her face, colour to her. She looked so grey that first day she took Noah to see me, like life had washed out of her. But there's something there now.

And her tits are massive.

I don't think we'll ever be really close friends. I think we've done too much to each other for that.

But we won't be cruel. We will help when needed and let each other be and smile, and say nice things to each other and about each other.

She drops Scout off for playdates sometimes, if the kids nag. Sometimes I take Noah round there, leave him with them. It feels like a second home to him, after he stayed.

And it means I get some time to write.

I'm only a few chapters in, but Callum reckons the new book will be better.

'There are so many books like *The Women Who Watch On*,' he said, 'that could be written any time. Write this while it's fresh.'

I'm treating this one like a kind of therapy, but he's said he wants it, based on what he's seen. This one is about women and the dark things we do to each other in the underbelly of the internet.

This one isn't about someone made up, it's about me.

AFTERWORD

What happens when a human becomes a platform? A one-person brand manipulated by an algorithm that feeds anxiety, comparison and insecurity: an app that wants you to be your best authentic self while only showing a highlights reel of your life?

I've read things that paint a ghoulish picture of those trying to make the most of 'these little squares' and others that place them on a pedestal. Both versions I find troubling. Other than, perhaps, Greta Thunberg and Fred West, no person is inherently good or bad. People don't fit into boxes and there's so much greyness and nuance that gets lost. How can you show all the complexities of a human in a photo with 200-word caption? It's flat, binary and 2D. You're left with a polished fragment of a person.

So with this book, we wanted to delve into the complexity of female friendships under the glare of a smartphone: what can be a heady cocktail of support and envy, joy and judgement, dopamine highs and lows, all mixed up with post-natal depression or unresolved trauma and the thousand other stresses that we live with every day.

It mattered that Lo and Dyl were strong yet flawed women united by the innocence of their children and the weight of motherhood. United by the loneliness, the desperation to give everything to your child while managing the loss of identity, friends, jobs and, in turn, perspective.

And to challenge what 'women supporting women' really means. I don't blindly support every woman I meet, because feminism isn't a cult. But I do believe in raising up where you can and that we don't need to tear each other down.

Because the one thing I do know is that cancelling someone online can cancel them offline too.

This novel is for everyone who is more than one thing.

Anna
London, 2021

ACKNOWLEDGEMENTS

Firstly, we'd like to thank our families, for making us who we are (for good and bad).

Thanks to Charlotte Mursell for seeing what this book was hoping to be and helping us make it so, along with Olivia Barber and the whole Orion team.

Thanks to Abi Bergstrom, Megan Staunton and Gleam Titles.

Also our early readers, in particular Georgia, Gemma, Bella, Hersha and El (who deserves extra credit for the Pommes de Terre de Toms).

Thanks to Deborah Baxter and Melissa Kelly at The Modern Family Law Company for their patience with our doubtlessly dim questions about UK family law.

And thanks to the many hundreds of people who have offered kind words and considered criticism on the more open corners of the internet for the last five years.

Matt Farquharson
Anna Whitehouse
London, 2021

CREDITS

Anna Whitehouse, Matt Farquharson and Orion Fiction would like to thank everyone at Orion who worked on the publication of *Underbelly* in the UK.

Editorial
Charlotte Mursell
Sanah Ahmed

Copy editor
Emily Thomas

Proof reader
Jade Craddock

Audio
Paul Stark

Contracts
Anne Goddard

Production
Ruth Sharvell

Design
Rabab Adams
Joanna Ridley
Nick May

Editorial Management
Charlie Panayiotou
Jane Hughes
Alice Davis

Finance
Jasdip Nandra
Afeera Ahmed
Elizabeth Beaumont
Sue Baker

Marketing
Helena Fouracre